BRAIN TRAINING
the complete **visual** program

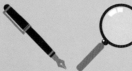

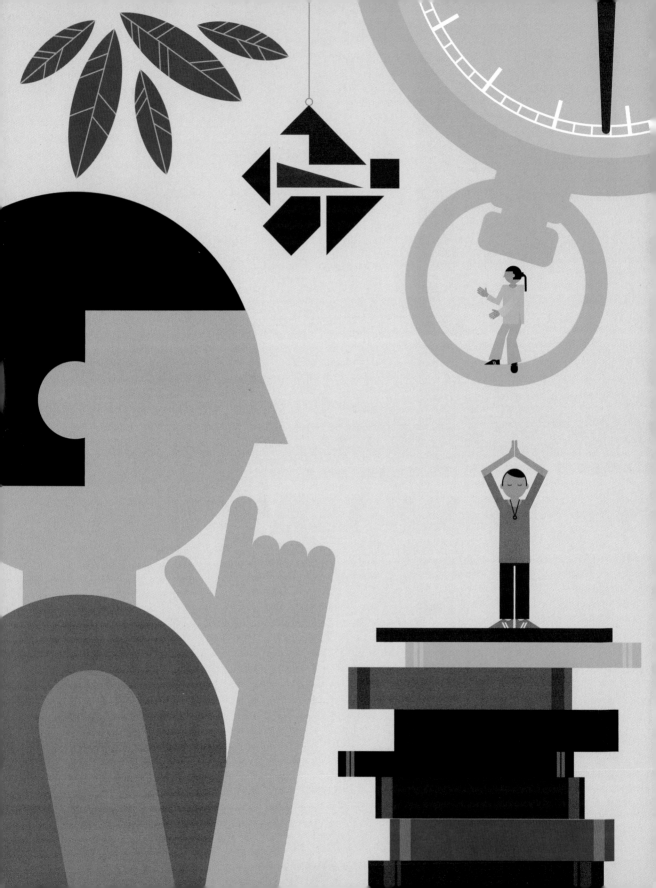

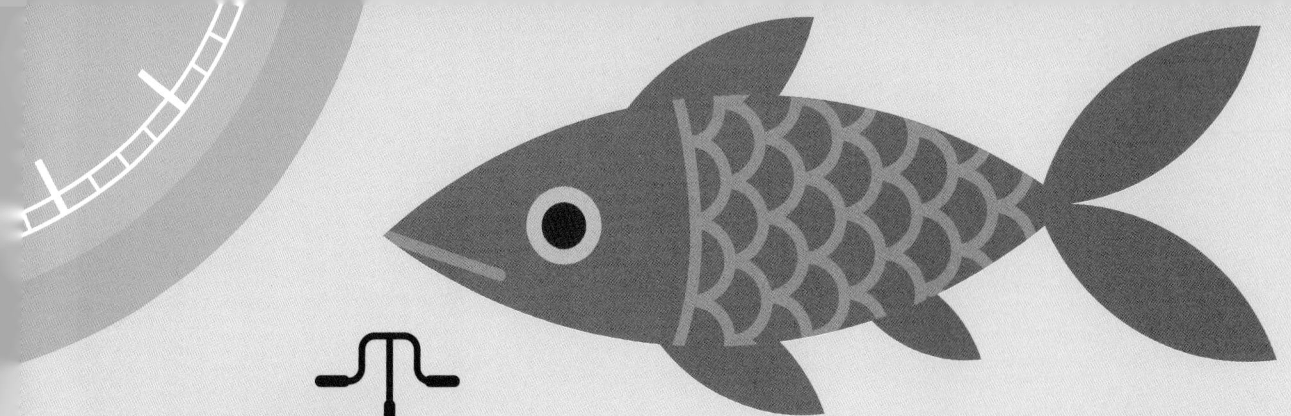

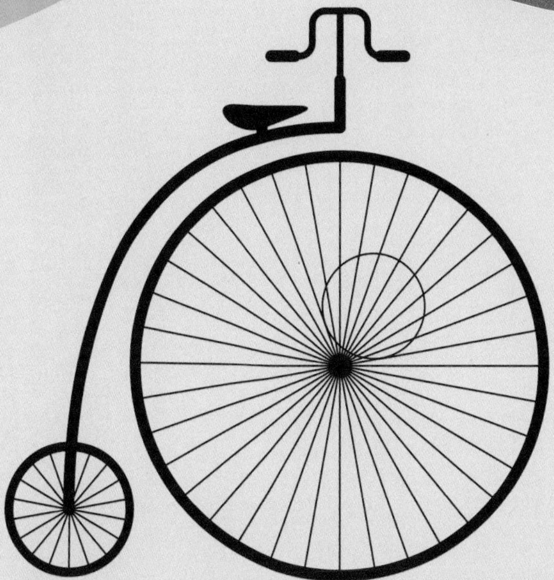

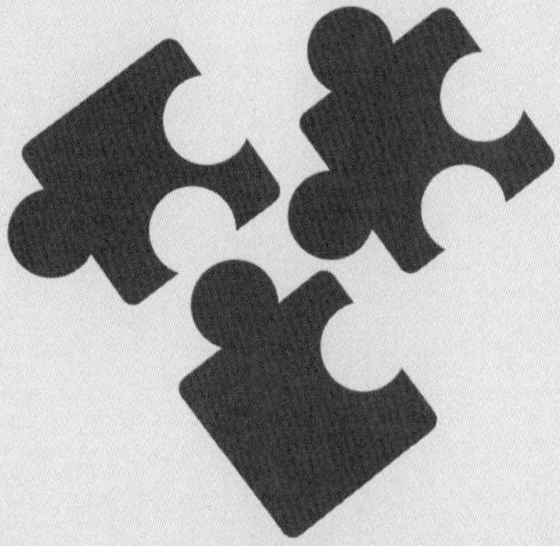

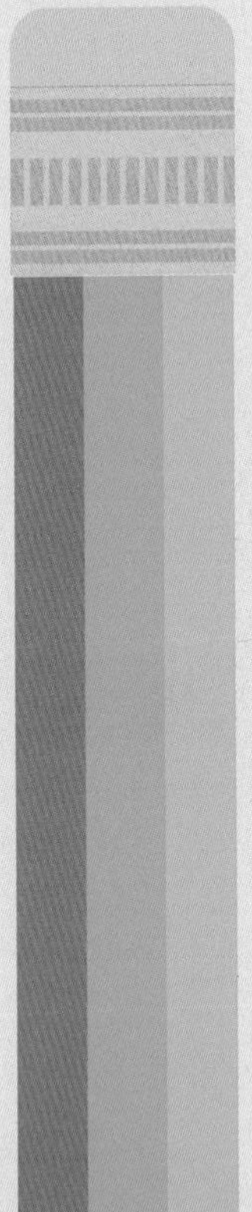

BRAIN TRAINING
the complete **visual** program

foreword by **Tony Buzan**

written by **James Harrison** and **Mike Hobbs**

DK

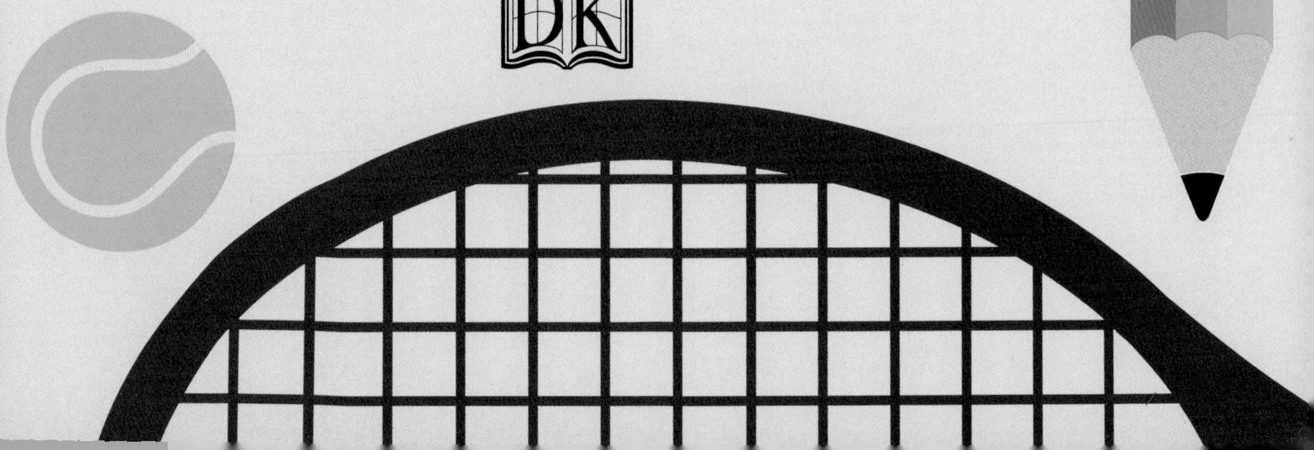

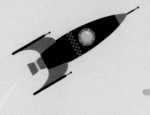

LONDON, NEW YORK, MUNICH, MELBOURNE, DELHI

Illustrator & Designer Keith Hagan at
www.greenwich-design.co.uk
Project Editor Suhel Ahmed
Project Art Editor Charlotte Seymour
Senior Editor Helen Murray
US Editors Shannon Beatty, Jill Hamilton and
Margaret Parrish
Senior Art Editor Liz Sephton
Senior Production Editor Jennifer Murray
Production Controller Alice Holloway
Creative Technical Support Sonia Charbonnier
Managing Editor Penny Warren
Managing Art Editors Glenda Fisher and
Marianne Markham
Category Publisher Peggy Vance
Puzzles Consultant Phil Chambers

The authors and publishers have made every effort to acknowledge the relevant puzzle and quiz providers and to ensure that the external websites are correct and active at the time of going to press.

Published in the United States by DK Publishing
375 Hudson Street, New York, New York 10014

10 11 12   10 9 8 7 6 5 4 3 2 1

A catalog record for this book is available from the Library of Congress.
ISBN: 978-0-7566-5730-7

DK books are available at special discounts when purchased in bulk for sales promotions, premiums, fund-raising, or educational use. For details, contact: DK Publishing Special Markets, 375 Hudson Street, New York, New York 10014 or SpecialSales@dk.com.

Printed and bound in Singapore by Star Standard
Discover more at **www.dk.com**

Contents

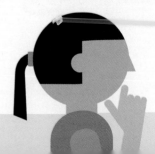

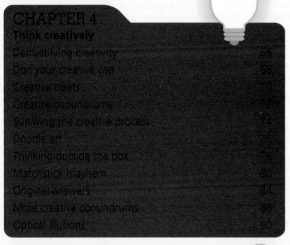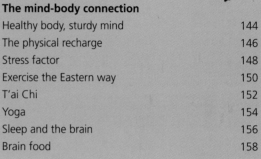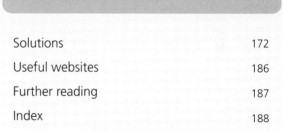
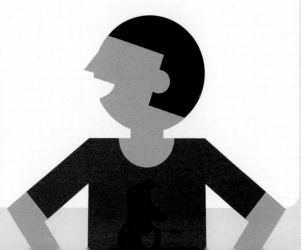

→ Foreword

It is the dream of everyone to have a brain that works better. You are holding in your hands a book that will help you make that dream come true!

Brain Training is one of the first VISUAL guides to enhancing your mental acumen. In this New Age of Intelligence, in which the human brain has to think intelligently about managing knowledge and processing the information it is bombarded with, it's vitally important that learning materials are brain-friendly. One of the reasons I was so enthusiastic about writing the foreword for *Brain Training* is that this book has everything your brain needs: it is written in the brain's own language—the "visual" language. It contains relevant images, plentiful color, excellent spatial design, clear associations, and lucid writing. It is a book about the brain that is friendly to the brain. In its physical form, the book is entirely congruent with what the brain needs.

In maximizing your brain it is also important for you to know that, for learning, the majority of people do not use their full cognitive potential. This might sound like bad news, but is actually good news. It means that you have a lot of untapped brainpower still left in the tank. All you need to do is learn how to access it! *Brain Training* will allow you to do that, by introducing you to exciting and enjoyable games and exercises that will help you maximize your intelligence.

In this groundbreaking book, you will learn about your brain and its remarkable structure and capacity. You will also be enlightened about the power of your visual and imaginative processes. You will find out about your memory and its extraordinary capacities, your innate visual and creative capabilities, and your ability with numbers. The book will

offer "visual" approaches to increase your verbal reasoning and word power. There is also a chapter that addresses the vitally important relationship between your brain and your body, and in which you will learn that the ancient adage: "Healthy Body Healthy Mind, Healthy Mind Healthy Body" is true. By working through the puzzles in *Brain Training*, you will improve your focus and concentration, your memory, and your learning and creative powers. These are abilities that will significantly boost your confidence and joy in life.

By investing in the *Brain Training* program, you have invested in your own intellectual capital, and that capital is the most valuable capital in the world.

Tony Buzan,
Inventor of Mind Maps®

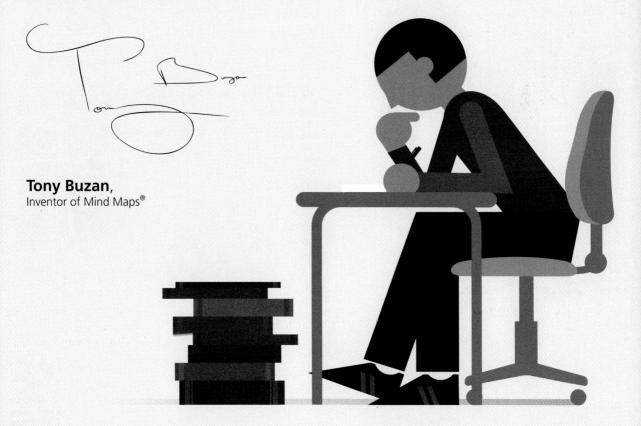

How to use this book

Studies show that the sense of sight is the most receptive when it comes to learning. Therefore, this program is visually led, and is filled with a diverse mix of popular cognitive exercises, which are divided into thematic chapters covering memory, visual reasoning and spatial awareness, creativity, numeracy, verbal reasoning, and the mind-body connection.

We open with a general introduction to the brain, and to the concept of intelligence and visual learning. This is followed by a range of exercises—"Where are you at?"—to gauge your current mental agility. In the subsequent chapters we concentrate on a specific brain function, such as memory or creativity. First, we explain how it works and then we offer the most effective puzzles to exercise that particular mental function.

Working through the book

The structure allows you to either work through the book from cover to cover or to pick out a specific topic—for example, memory—and work on it alone. However you choose to approach the book, we encourage you to start with the first chapter (and the "Where are you at?" exercises) and finish with the final workout in Chapter 8, so you can gauge how you have improved over time.

For the majority of exercises we have provided answer boxes for you to fill in. For the remaining exercises, we will instruct you to write your answer on a separate sheet of paper. Finally, in "The mind-body connection" chapter, we will introduce you to the type of foods, exercise, and other physical pick-me-ups that raise brain power.

Technique pages offer tips and strategies for improving brain function

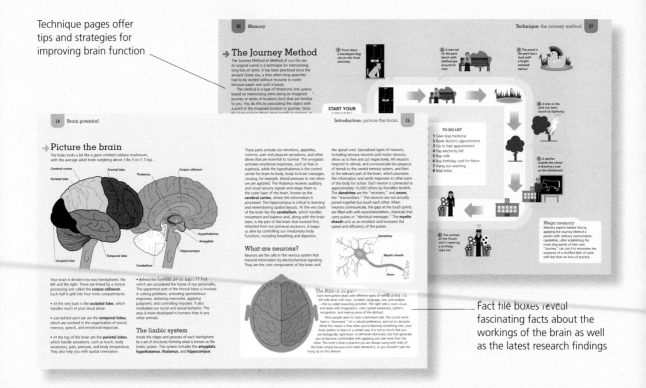

Fact file boxes reveal fascinating facts about the workings of the brain as well as the latest research findings

Hints and strategies

We also include techniques throughout the book, such as "The Journey Method" (see p.36) for improving memory or "The physical recharge" (see p.146) to increase mental alertness. These appear as discrete features between exercises, and come complete with an example of how and why you might use the technique. We encourage you to learn and apply these to the relevant exercises in the chapter. We might prompt you to use a specific technique to complete an exercise so that you become familiar with applying it, which is an important part of improving your brainpower. Also, try to learn the hints and tips we offer throughout the book (denoted by the lightning strike icon), as these will enhance your ability to

work with the material. There are also "fact file" boxes, which offer fascinating information about the workings of the brain.

You can use all the tips and techniques you have learned to complete the mix of exercises in the final workout (Chapter 8). You may then want to return to the start and retest yourself against the puzzles in the "Where are you at?" section to assess overall improvement.

Solutions

Finally, you can find the solutions and/or explanations to the puzzles at the back of the book. Look for the solutions arrow at the foot of the page, which guides you to the specific page number.

The colored band at the top of the page indicates puzzle pages

Answer boxes to fill in as you work through the puzzles

Top tip boxes are indicated by a lightning strike icon

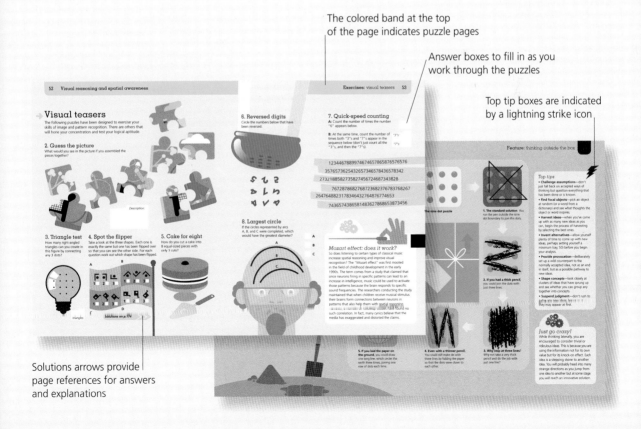

Solutions arrows provide page references for answers and explanations

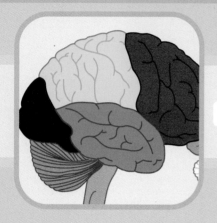
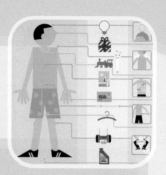
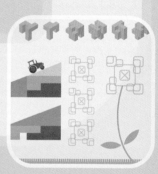
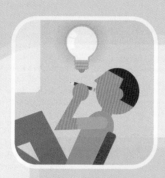
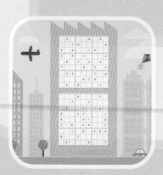
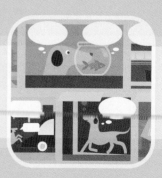

Chapter 1
Brain potential

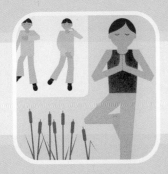

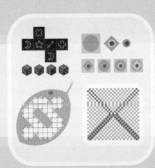

→ Brain power

Your brain is the most sophisticated object in the known universe. Millions of messages are speeding through your nervous system at any given moment, enabling your brain to receive, process, and store information, and to send instructions all over the body.

Your brain is capable of so much more than you might give it credit for. Just take a moment to consider all the things made by human beings. From the earliest tool, such as a pickax, to the modern skyscraper, and from the largest dam to the smallest microchip—the human brain is where all of these objects were first conceived. Undoubtedly, the brain is the most powerful tool at mankind's disposal.

Your brain works around the clock. It generates more electrical impulses each day than all the mobile phones in the world. You have billions of tiny brain nerve cells interacting with each other in permutations that have been estimated to equal 1 with 800 zeros behind it. (To make that remotely graspable, the number of atoms in the world—one of the smallest material things we can get a fix on— is estimated to be 1.33 with 48 zeros after it.)

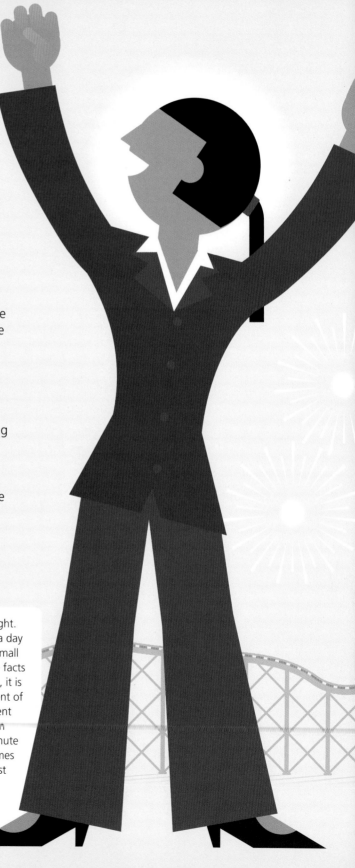

Did you know?

Your brain runs on less power than your refrigerator light. That's about 12 watts of power. During the course of a day your brain uses the amount of energy contained in a small chocolate bar, around 230 calories. Even though these facts might make the brain sound efficient, in relative terms, it is an energy hog. Your brain accounts for merely 2 percent of the body's weight, but consumes 20 percent of the body's total energy. Your brain requires a tenth of a calorie per minute merely to survive. Your brain consumes energy at ten times the rate of the rest of the body per gram of tissue. The majority of this energy goes into maintenance of the brain.

Strengths and weaknesses

So, if we have such a powerful brain, why aren't we all good at everything? Why are some of us forgetful? Why do some of us have trouble reading maps? Why do some of us lack a sense of rhythm? Surely with all that "electrical" activity going on inside our heads, we shouldn't be faced with these difficulties?

Think of the brain as a busy fairground with an assortment of rides and attractions, each representing a different area of the brain, and think of the people as the tiny nerve cells or "neurons" (see p.15). Now, the popularity of the various attractions tends to differ from one fairground to another; a ride in one fairground may draw more people than the same ride in another. In brain terms, the "popular rides" are the parts of the brain with lots of "nerve cell" activity and, hence, tend to be more developed. This development is aided significantly by the kind of education we receive as a child. One person

can be proficient when it comes to reading maps, another might be more creative, and a third, more logical. Of course, this is a crude analogy because the different areas of the brain function together for most tasks and a specific area dominates, but it does illustrate how the brain differs from person to person. In short, it's a question of education and genetics. So, don't be too hard on yourself if you think you're bad at math or terrible at languages. The chances are that you excel in another area.

However, this doesn't mean you cannot develop a mental ability that you consider weaker than another. It's wrong to think that just because you're not naturally gifted in something, such as math or map-reading, that there's no point in trying to improve it. Your brain is similar to any muscle in your body in that exercise will raise its potency. You can always strive to improve and expand your current mental aptitude.

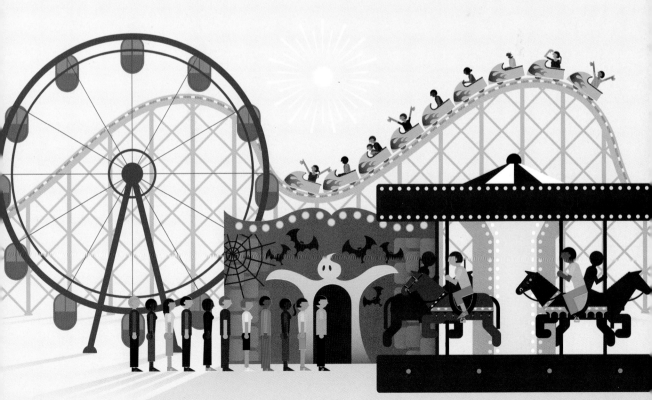

Picture the brain

The brain looks a bit like a giant crinkled rubbery mushroom, with the average adult brain weighing about 3 lbs 5 oz (1.5 kg).

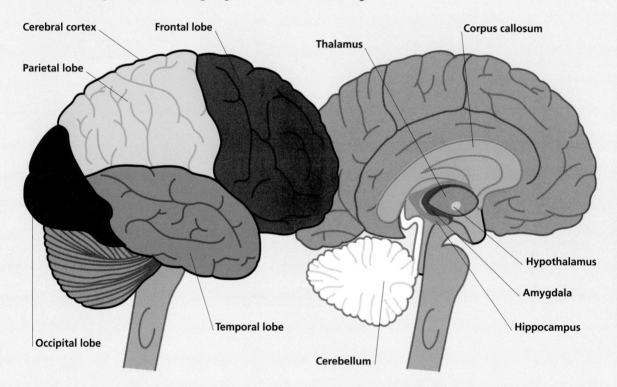

Cerebral cortex **Frontal lobe** **Thalamus** **Corpus callosum**

Parietal lobe

Hypothalamus

Amygdala

Hippocampus

Temporal lobe

Occipital lobe

Cerebellum

Your brain is divided into two hemispheres: the left and the right. These are linked by a central processing unit called the **corpus callosum**. Each half is split into four more compartments:

• At the very back is the **occipital lobe,** which handles much of your visual sense.

• Just behind each ear are the **temporal lobes**, which are involved in the organization of sound, memory, speech, and emotional responses.

• At the top of the brain are the **parietal lobes**, which handle sensations, such as touch, body awareness, pain, pressure, and body temperature. They also help you with spatial orientation.

• Behind the forehead are the **frontal lobes**, which are considered the home of our personality. The uppermost part of the frontal lobes is involved in solving problems, activating spontaneous responses, retrieving memories, applying judgment, and controlling impulses. It also modulates our social and sexual behavior. This area is more developed in humans than in any other animals.

The limbic system

Inside the ridges and grooves of each hemisphere lie a set of structures forming what is known as the limbic system. This system includes the **amygdala**, **hypothalamus**, **thalamus**, and **hippocampus**.

These parts activate our emotions, appetites, instincts, pain and pleasure sensations, and other drives that are essential to survival. The amygdala activates emotional responses, such as fear or euphoria, while the hypothalamus is the control center for brain-to-body, body-to-brain messages, causing, for example, blood pressure to rise when we are agitated. The thalamus receives auditory and visual sensory signals and relays them to the outer layer of the brain, known as the **cerebral cortex**, where the information is processed. The hippocampus is critical to learning and remembering spatial layouts. At the very back of the brain lies the **cerebellum**, which handles movement and balance and, along with the brain stem, is the part of the brain that evolved first, inherited from our primeval ancestors. It keeps us alive by controlling our involuntary body functions, including breathing and digestion.

What are neurons?

Neurons are the cells in the nervous system that transmit information by electrochemical signaling. They are the core components of the brain and the spinal cord. Specialized types of neurons, including sensory neurons and motor neurons, allow us to feel and act respectively. All neurons respond to stimuli, and communicate the presence of stimuli to the central nervous system, and then to the relevant part of the brain, which processes the information and sends responses to other parts of the body for action. Each neuron is connected to approximately 10,000 others by frondlike tendrils. The **dendrites** are the "receivers," and **axons**, the "transmitters." The neurons are not actually joined together but touch each other. When neurons communicate, the gaps at the touch points are filled with with neurotransmitters, chemicals that carry pulses or "electrical messages." The **myelin sheath** acts as an insulator and increases the speed and efficiency of the pulses.

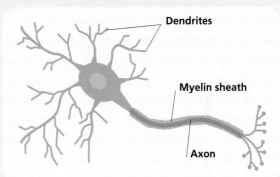

Dendrites

Myelin sheath

Axon

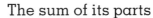

The sum of its parts

Each hemisphere deals with different types of mental activity. The left side deals with logic, numbers, language, lists, and analysis —the so-called reasoning activities. The right side is more visual, and deals with imagination, color, spatial awareness, pattern, recognition, and making sense of the abstract.

Most people seem to have a dominant side. The crucial word here is "dominant." It's a natural preference, and not an absolute. What this means is that when you're learning something new, your brain prefers to learn in a certain way. It is not so much that you are biologically right-brain- or left-brain-dominant, but that generally you've become comfortable with applying one side more than the other. The truth is that in practice you are always using both sides of the brain simply because most tasks demand it, so you shouldn't get too hung up on this division.

What is intelligence?

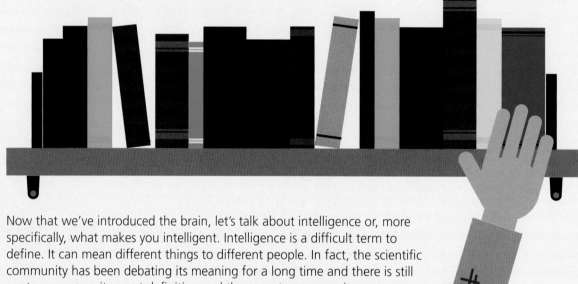

Now that we've introduced the brain, let's talk about intelligence or, more specifically, what makes you intelligent. Intelligence is a difficult term to define. It can mean different things to different people. In fact, the scientific community has been debating its meaning for a long time and there is still controversy over its exact definition and the ways to measure it.

The "IQ" test was once regarded as the best way to measure intelligence. However, there is now a general awareness of its shortcomings, namely, that it only tests specific branches of intelligence (see opposite). The important thing to bear in mind is that being intelligent is not only about excelling in a narrow academic field, or having a broad general knowledge, or even being good at spelling or math. All those things require a degree of intelligence but do not define intelligence. Rather, intelligence reflects a broader and deeper aptitude for understanding multiple things in one's surroundings, for catching on, making sense of things, or figuring out what to do in any given circumstance. It's about possessing the ability to analyze and evaluate, to imagine and invent, and, in practical terms, being able to apply and implement ideas successfully.

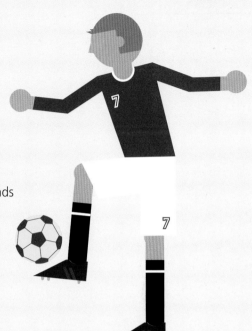

Strands of intelligence

There are innumerable strands of intelligence, such as the capacities to reason, plan, solve problems, think abstractly, comprehend ideas, use language, and learn. People's intelligence may also be characterized by their ability to adapt to a new environment, or their ability to form healthy relationships, or their capacity for original and productive thought. Furthermore, one could point out more specific strands of intelligence. For example, a person who excels in a specific sport is demonstrating a high level of kinesthetic intelligence, whereas a person who can manipulate melody and rhythm has high musical intelligence. In that respect, both Johann Sebastian Bach and David Beckham could be regarded as highly intelligent people in their respective fields.

The IQ test

IQ is the acronym for *intelligence quotient*, and refers to a score given for several standardized intelligence tests. French psychologist Alfred Binet developed the first of these in 1905. He constructed the IQ test, as it would later be called, to determine which children might need additional help in scholarly pursuits. The modern-day IQ test is primarily based on three intelligences: verbal reasoning, numerical reasoning, and visual-spatial reasoning. The system scores you on your understanding of everyday words, simple arithmetical concepts, and the ability to recognize shapes and interpret representational pictures.

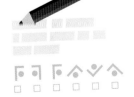

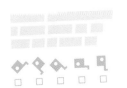

Brain training and intelligence

According to research carried out by the University of Michigan, a good brain-training program can improve working memory and boost general problem-solving ability, which can raise general intelligence. In the study, after recording the subjects' mental agility in a variety of cognitive tests, the researchers gave the subjects a series of brain-training exercises. This mental workout was given to four groups, who repeated the exercises for 8, 12, 17, or 19 days. After the training the researchers retested the subjects' intelligence. Although the performance of the untrained group improved marginally, the trained subjects showed a significant improvement, which increased with the amount of time spent training. This suggests that a good brain-training program is an effective way to boost intelligence.

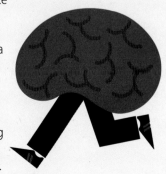

Looking to learn

How much do you learn from your sense of sight? Well, in general, most experts agree that about 75 percent of your learning is through your visual sense. Take babies, for instance. With their inquisitive eyes they pick up behavior traits by observing the things that people do around them; they process and interpret facial expressions and physical gestures. From a single glance, babies can tell when their mothers are happy or angry with them. It's not something that ever changes. Consider two people who go out on a first date. How much attention are they really paying to the conversation and how much attention are they spending on reading each other's body language?

The fact that you pick up a great deal of information from sight isn't surprising since about 40 percent of your brain is dedicated to seeing and processing visual material. On average, most people know the names of approximately 10,000 objects and can recognize them by their shapes alone.

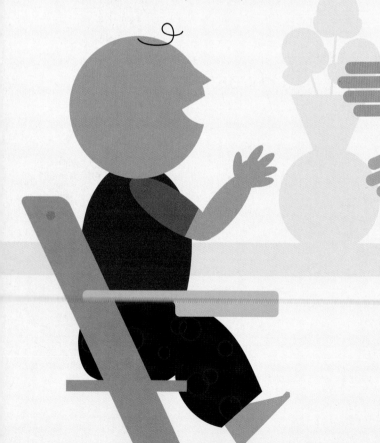

Visual sense

Your visual sense is key to interacting with the world around you. By the time most children are six years old, it is estimated that they've already committed to memory the names of a fifth of the objects they will know in their lifetime. Studies have shown that visual stimulation helps brain development the most, and aids more sophisticated types of learning both when you're growing up and during adulthood.

The ability to glean information from more abstract types of visuals, such as tables, graphs, webs, maps, and illustrations, is unique to the human race. By being able to interpret information from such sources, you are able to find meaning, reorganize and group similar things, and compare and analyze disparate information. In learning, your visual sense is undoubtedly the most useful and widely used.

Taking instruction

The amazing thing about the visual part of your brain is that once it sees something a certain way, it tries to develop a memory of it. For example, if you're trying to learn a dance sequence from watching someone else perform, your brain will collect the visual information, process it, and then try to memorize it. You can then use the memory to practice and develop proficiency. Let's stimulate your visual sense to learn something new.

Seeing is believing

Try this. What do you see in the image below?
    Of course, it's a maple leaf—the motif of the Canadian flag. But look again. Can you see the two men who are clearly riled, and head-butting each other? Look closely. Their faces are formed by the outline of the top half of the leaf. The men have very pointed noses.
    From now on, every time you see the Canadian flag, your mind's eye will flit between the picture of the maple leaf and the two angry men. You tend to learn more when your preconceptions have been challenged. If you see something you think you recognize but it turns out to be something else, that's memorable.

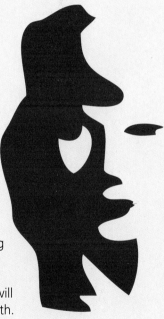

Take a look at the image on the right. What do you see: the face of a young woman or a saxophonist playing his instrument? If you study the picture for long enough, eventually you will be able to see both images, and your brain will develop a memory of both.

A visual guide

The puzzles and exercises throughout the book have a strong visual element. Following this principle, you will find that the brain-training program provides you with a constant interplay between words and images. This synergy will help you exercise your cognitive muscles the most. In fact, one study showed that those who used visual presentation tools to convey information were 43 percent more successful than those who did not.

Where are you at?

Welcome to the *Brain Training* program. Before we introduce you to some of the tips and techniques for improving various mental faculties, let's find out your current mental agility.

The following exercises will introduce you to the type of brain workout that will primarily stimulate your visual sense, but we've also included some nonvisual tests to provide a contrast. You'll be given a score for each exercise you complete. Add up the score at the end to find out your current cognitive aptitude.

1. Home and away

A: Try to memorize these 9 simple landmarks in order in 1 minute. Then cover them up and see how many you can remember.

Grand Canyon
Eiffel Tower
Statue of Liberty
Taj Mahal
Acropolis
Niagara Falls
Egyptian Pyramids
Great Wall of China
Mount Rushmore

B: Now try to memorize these 9 household objects in order in 1 minute. Then cover them up and see how many you can remember.

Window	Radio
Toothbrush	Wastebasket
Book	Magazine
Frame	Plate
Cup	

•1–3 = 1 point
•4–6 = 2 points
•7+ = 3 points

•1–3 = 1 point
•4–6 = 2 points
•7+ = 3 points

2. Number sequences

Work out the next number in each of the following sequences.

A: 3, 12, 48, 192

B: 1, 1, 2, 3, 5, 8

C: 2, 5, 10, 17, 26

D: 5, 13, 29, 61, 125

•A: 2 points
•B: 2 points
•C: 3 points
•D: 3 points

Solutions on p.172

3. Building fences

Which pile of sticks was used to create the fence?

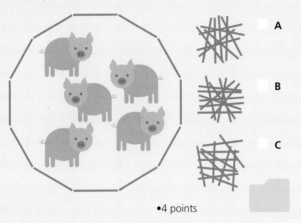

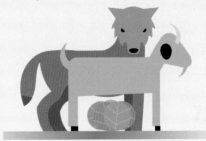

A

B

C

•4 points

4. Goat, cabbage, and wolf

A farmer needs to ferry a goat, a cabbage, and a wolf across a river. Besides the farmer himself, the boat allows him to carry only one of them at a time. Without supervision, the goat will gobble up the cabbage and the wolf will not hesitate to feast on the goat. How can he ferry all of them safely to the other side?

•4 points

5. Mental arithmetic

Complete this set of mental arithmetic questions in the fastest time possible.

A: 12 – 3 =

B: 9 + 8 =

C: 2 x 10 =

D: 36 ÷ 3 =

E: 7 x 7 =

F: 8 x 4 =

G: 11 – 6 =

H: 9 x 8 =

I: 6 x 7 =

J: 9 + 7 =

K: 17 – 8 =

L: 14 – 5 =

M: 5 x 8 =

N: 3 + 9 =

O: 4 x 6 =

•Under 20 secs = 3 points
•21–40 secs = 2 points
•41+ secs = 1 points

6. A perfect circle?

Is the inner shape a perfect circle, or just a little warped? Look closely.

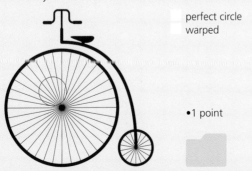

perfect circle
warped

•1 point

Novelty factor

What makes good mental stimulation? The answer is challenge, novelty, and variety. Don't do only numerical exercises because that will only stimulate your number-crunching skills, and if you concentrate only on crosswords, it will fire up only your aptitude for language. And if you only look at words and numbers, that won't spark your visual and spatial awareness. Returning to the fairground metaphor (see p.13), it is a case of activating every ride, not just the ones that you are good at or like the most.

7. Personal diary

Write down two specific things you did ...

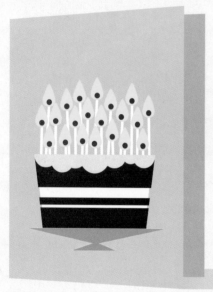

Note: you're not allowed to write the same things.

A: Yesterday

B: Same day last week

C: Same day a month ago

D: On your last birthday

• A: 1 point for each thing you remember
• B: 2 points for each thing you remember
• C: 3 points for each thing you remember
• D: 1 point for each thing you remember

8. Dog and bone

Divide the square into four identical sections, so that in each section there is a dog with a bone. One dog will not have a bone because he's suffering from a toothache.

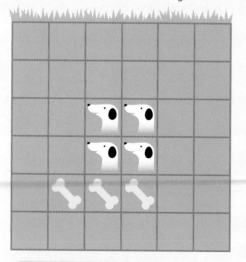

• 4 points

9. Light switches

Three light switches control 3 lights upstairs. When you click the switches you cannot see which switch controls which light. You know that all the lights are off when the switches are up. You are allowed just one visit upstairs, then you have to say which switch matches which light. How can you do it?

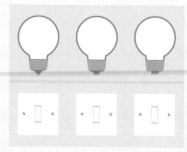

• 3 points

Solutions on p.172 ⟫

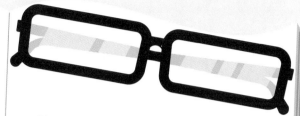

10. Speed reading

Read out loud the following passage as fast as you can and try to articulate every word.

Examining how you react in a given situation might be a useful way to understand thoughts and feelings you find difficult to put into words. It might give you an insight into your own deeper motives, and enlighten you to personal anxieties and frailties that you might have not been conscious of before.

You can access these emotions by creating or finding a story or parable that is clearly fictional, but nevertheless has some parallels to a real situation you are facing. Ideally, you would read it to yourself (or you could draw your own picture, whichever you prefer doing).

If you choose to create your own, you don't have to be a good drawer or writer (stick figure drawings or amateur narration would suffice). It isn't necessary for anyone else to see or read your work, although it is usually more productive if you can get someone else's perspective or reaction.

Because the story or picture is not a description of your actual situation, you are at liberty to be creative—you can make things happen as you wish them to; you can present things in particular ways just because they "feel right." You can note what has to happen for you to feel comfortable.

You are definitely not saying that "this is what will happen under these circumstances," but you are holding it up as a mirror to yourself, and noting the sorts of beliefs, expectations, feelings, judgments, and anxieties that you may well find yourself bringing to such a situation.

Putting something into this framework makes it easier to describe your concern to others, and may increase the range of metaphors and images you can naturally use when talking to others.

Should some areas of the story summon strong negative feelings, this may suggest a need for finding positive ways to handle similar feelings in the real situation for instance, getting a colleague to help you out in situations you may not handle too well. Similarly, if you find yourself being judgmental or negative about someone in your story, you may need to develop ways to see such people more compassionately.

In time, you may become aware of cultural assumptions and expectations—what "ought" or "ought not" to happen by your (but perhaps not other people's) conventions.

- Under 1 min 20 secs = 3 points
- 1 min 20 – 1 min 40 secs = 2 points
- Over 1 min 40 secs = 1 point

Benefits of reading aloud

Modern brain-scanning techniques such as fMRI (functional Magnetic Resonance Imaging) have revealed that reading aloud lights up many areas of the brain in both hemispheres. There is intense activity in areas associated with articulation and hearing the sound of the spoken response, which strengthens the connective structures of your brain cells for more brainpower. This leads to an overall improvement in concentration. Reading aloud is also a good way to develop your oratory skills because it forces you to read each and every word—something people don't often do when skimming, or reading in silence. Children, in particular, should be encouraged to read aloud because the brain is wired for learning through connections that are created by positive stimulation, such as singing, touching, and reading aloud.

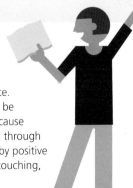

11. Spot the difference

Study the picture on the left for 30 seconds. Then cover it up and circle the 6 alterations made to the same picture on the right.

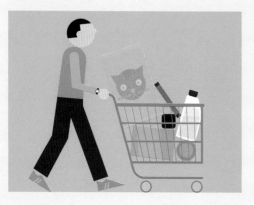

- •1–2 differences
    = 1 point

- •3–4 differences
    = 2 points

- •5–6 differences
    = 3 points

12. Numerical jigsaw

The vertical strips below each contain 4 numbers or symbols. Rearrange these **strips** in the quickest time possible so that 4 valid equations appear across the rows. In each equation, operations are done horizontally. Write the correct answers in the grid provided.

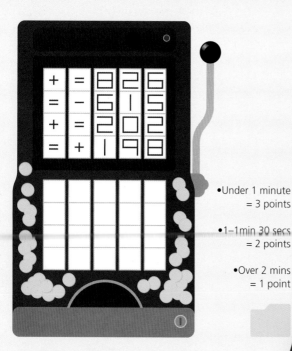

- •Under 1 minute
    = 3 points

- •1–1min 30 secs
    = 2 points

- •Over 2 mins
    = 1 point

13. Visual logic test

Look at the set of pictures below. Which one doesn't belong in each group?

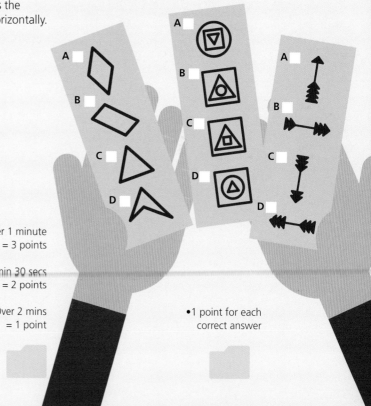

- •1 point for each
    correct answer

14. Manhole covers

Why is it better to have round manhole covers than square ones? Look at the picture and think about it. It's not a trick question. There is more than one answer.

•2 points

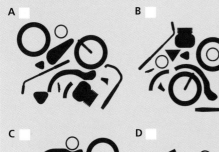

15. Moving by degrees

If the hour hand on a clock moves $\frac{1}{60}$th of a degree every minute, then how many degrees will the hour hand move in one hour?

•2 points

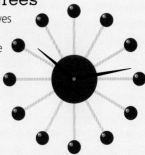

16. Motorcycle parts

Which of the four options has exactly the right parts to complete the motorcycle?

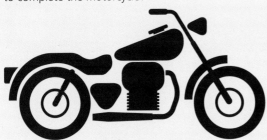

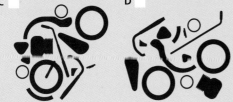

A   B

C   D

Solutions on p.172   •3 points

17. Straight lines?

Are the two horizontal lines straight or curved?

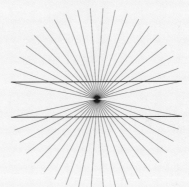

straight
curved

•1 point

Did you know?

Generally, it's accepted that brain function naturally starts to deteriorate once we get past our mid-20s. This is not unlike athletes being at their physical peak and then having to work harder to keep fit as they get older. The good news is that there's no need to worry. The size and weight of your brain remains roughly the same until you reach 90, providing that you keep it active. In fact, there's no reason to believe that you can't keep your brain lively throughout your life by giving it new experiences, challenges, tests, and puzzles. These improve cell connections so that your brain's overall function remains sound regardless of your age.

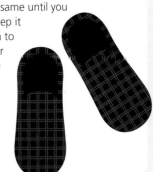

18. Abstract art

What you see on the right is the Rey-Osterrieth Complex Figure Test. Neurologists commonly use it to assess a patient's memory and attention span.

Look at the figure and copy it on a separate sheet of paper. This should help you memorize the details. Then cover up the original and the copy, and begin drawing it from memory on a piece of paper. You have 1 minute to draw as much of it as you can. How much of it can you recall?

•Quarter of it = 2 points
•Half of it = 3 points
•Two-thirds + = 5 points

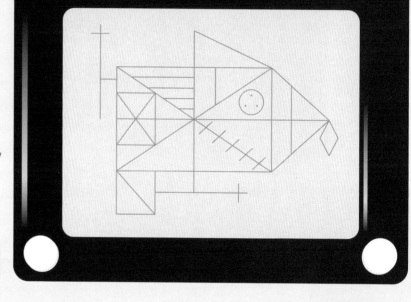

19. Magic square

The numbers in all rows, columns, and both diagonals of the grid add up to 15. You have to use the numbers 1 to 9; a number cannot be repeated. We've filled three squares. Fill in the missing numbers:

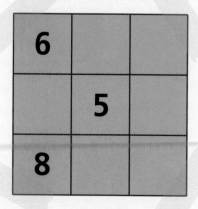

•Under 45 secs = 3 points
•45 secs −1 min = 2 points
•Over 1 mins = 1 point

20. Color mazes

Find a path from the bottom left to the top right that passes through an equal number of squares of each (nonwhite) color. To the right is a solved example.

Note: the line passes through two yellow squares, two red squares, and two blue squares.

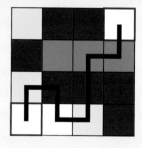

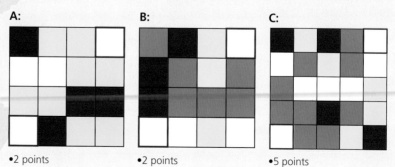

A: •2 points

B: •2 points

C: •5 points

21. A perfectly boiled egg

You want to boil an egg for 15 minutes. However, you have only a 7-minute and an 11-minute egg timer at your disposal. How can you ensure that you boil the egg for exactly 15 minutes using only these two timers? Write your answer down on a separate sheet of paper.

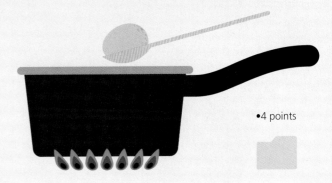

• 4 points

22. Spot the odd picture

In the list below, can you identify the picture that doesn't belong in each of the groups?

A

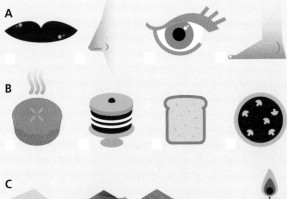

B

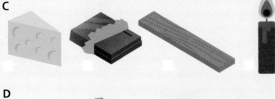

C

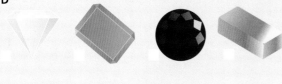

D

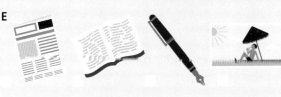

E

• 1 point for each correct answer

Solutions on p.173 ⟩⟩⟩

23. Odd word out

A	bear ☐	cat ☐	tiger ☐	dog ☐	fish ☐
B	stream ☐	pond ☐	lagoon ☐	lake ☐
C	cotton ☐	wood ☐	stool ☐	metal ☐
D	lawn ☐	thicket ☐	forest ☐	jungle ☐
E	Chepre ☐	Cyprus ☐	Corfu ☐	Zypern ☐

• 1 point for each correct answer

How did you do?

It's time to add up your points. Turn to pages 172 and 173 for the answers and figure out your score. There is a total of 100 points up for grabs.

YOUR SCORE: /100

How well have you done so far? Has your score impressed you? Did you perform well in some areas and moderately in others? That's only natural, because it's uncommon for a person to be equally good at numerical reasoning and verbal reasoning, for example. Bringing all your brain activities up to the level of their highest potential is what this book is for. Now continue to find out how to hone each mental faculty with tips, techniques, and more exercises.

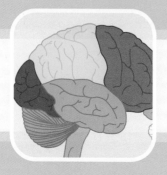

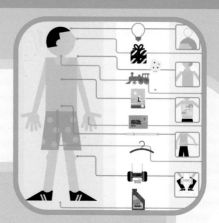

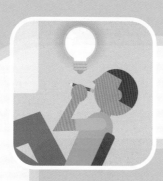

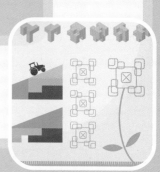

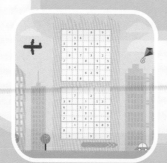

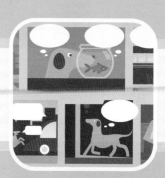

Chapter 2
Memory

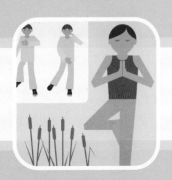

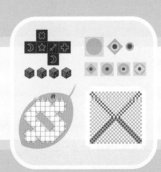

→ All about memory

Does our memory play tricks on us? It might seem so when we can vividly recount a happy or poignant episode from our childhood, yet fail to remember the name of someone we met only yesterday. Or we might be able to recall the entire lyrics of a song recorded by our favorite band, yet forget something as simple as which way to turn a screw to loosen it. Why is our memory selective? Is it because our memory has a limited capacity, and so, consequently, we somehow prioritize what information to keep and what to discard? If this is the case then is it possible to find ways of boosting our memory? Perhaps we should address these questions once we find out what memory actually is.

What is memory?

Memory forms a key component of your intelligence. Everything you learn in your lifetime is organized and stored in some way. The efficiency with which you access this information is what defines whether you have a good or bad memory.

Scientists have spent much time seeking the location in the brain where memories are stored, identifying the hippocampus and rhinal cortex as possible sites (see p.43). However, contrary to what many of us might think, the latest research suggests that memory cannot be pinned down to any single part of the brain. In fact, it's false to think of memory as a storage facility crammed with everything you have ever learned, and a place you delve inside when you want to retrieve a piece of information.

Memory isn't a place, it's an activity, an experience: when you remember something you are actually reconstructing it from details you consider important. Your memory is selective and interpretive, and the mechanisms driving it are spread throughout the brain. Two people who witness the same event can give entirely different accounts. In short, you remember more clearly what an event means to you than the actual details.

Can memory be boosted?

Absolutely! Memory can be exercised, improved, and nurtured. The information your memory retains is influenced by the meaning you attach to it. For example, you are more likely to remember something if it is linked to a personal experience or emotion. You can boost your memory by giving the information you wish to memorize stronger meaning and associations. Memory works by:
• making something memorable
• organizing and then storing that piece of memorable information
• retrieving it accurately at any given time.

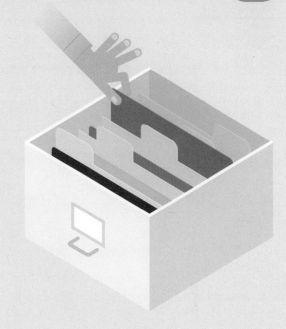

Memory myth

The myth we tend to hear most is that memory deteriorates as we get older. This is false. If the brain is stimulated regularly, it can actually improve with age. People in their 80s and 90s can possess the same memory power as people half their age. Brain cells don't die off as we get older. As

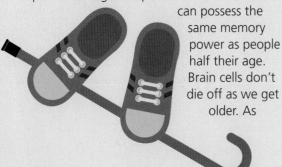

psychology author Tony Buzan reminds us: "senior moments are more to do with absent mindedness than absent memory." The best powers of recall do not necessarily belong to the young but to those who continue to hone their cognitive skills throughout life. Older people who engage in mentally taxing work, learn new skills, and keep physically active are likely to be in better mental shape than a younger person who doesn't do these things. Brain training offers a good cognitive workout. So here's your chance to exercise your brain and boost your memory. Turn over to learn some killer techniques.

The memory champs

At the annual World Memory Championships, contestants battle it out to see who has the best memory. In truth, these people are no smarter than you or me, they just take the time and make the effort to memorize information using a variety of mnemonics, or memory strategies (see p.33). For instance, by using the Journey Method (see p.36), memory champion, Ben Pridmore memorized a shuffled deck of playing cards in 26.28 seconds, beating the previous world record of 31.16 seconds set by Andi Bell. Two years earlier Dr. Gunther Karsten from Germany memorized a 1,949 digit number in an hour—and recalled it in under two hours. These guys prove what the memory is capable of if you apply the right techniques.

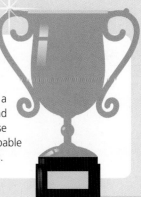

→ How does memory work?

Before we introduce you to the tips, let's look at three types of memory you possess to receive and keep track of information.

Sensory memory

You receive information from the senses, such as sight and hearing, and hold it for one or two seconds while you process it and decide what to do with it. What you ignore quickly fades and cannot be retrieved, much as sound dissolves. Remember how you can sometimes catch an echo of a sentence, or a glimpse of someone you sort of recognize when you're not really paying attention, but then, in an instant, it's gone.

Short-term memory

If you pay attention to something, the details are then transferred to the short-term memory, which can only store up to seven pieces of data at any one time. For instance, using this memory you can remember the digits of an internet bank account or a pin code for only as long as it takes for you to key it in. As soon as the short-term memory is "full," it only takes a new piece of information to dislodge an old one because the neural mechanisms, (the meanings and associations) have not been created to allow you to recall the information later on.

Some scientists believe that evolution has shaped this memory to have a limited capacity. Can you imagine if you were able to retain all the visual information you picked up in a day? What would happen if you kept a memory of every stranger you walked past and every sign you read? Well, your brain would eventually suffer from data overload. The advantage of a limited working memory is that it allows you to prioritize and focus on the task at hand.

Long-term memory

What makes information cross over to long-term memory? Any information can be committed to this memory through the process of rehearsal and meaningful association. Once processed, the information can be recalled weeks, months, or even years later. To make this effective, you must make as many links as possible to increase the number of starting points for retrieving the memory. Links are established when you cogitate, review, and analyze information. Association, in particular, relies on your visual memory (demonstrated with the Journey Method on p.36), which is an effective way of recalling a list of disparate items. One thing we do know about memory is that if it is linked to a personal experience or emotion it is more likely to be recalled. If you're not convinced, then think of a birthday. Which do you remember: your 10th, 15th, 18th, or 21st? Chances are it's your 18th or 21st because of the significance.

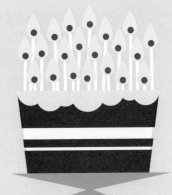

Memory aids

• **Association/Visualization:** the process of forming mental connections is what our brain naturally does to make sense of things. Information can be recalled more easily if you can relate it to an idea or object that you are familiar with (association), or if you can create a mental picture of it, as with Mind Maps (see p.62).

• **Review:** without review, most people can only recall about 20 percent of selected material after a 24-hour period. Students can significantly improve their learning by simply reviewing material once after class to clarify and confirm what they have heard, and once again later that day or evening. Reviewing material regularly will transfer information to your long-term memory.

• **Explanation:** of all memory techniques, "explanation" works best. When possible, put things into your own words. The combination of having the idea in your head and the words to express it is synergistic, creating a better understanding of the information, and significantly improving your ability to recall it.

• **Order:** the brain is very good at finding patterns and thinking to an order. The numbers 7 1 9 3 11 5 might seem hard to remember, but reorder them to 1 3 5 7 9 11 and it becomes much easier because the brain spots the sequence order instantly.

• **Senses:** use more of your senses than just sight: engage hearing, smell, taste, and touch to process information and make the memory trace stronger and longer-lasting.

• **Mnemonics:** it is easier for your memory to recall information if you create rhymes, sentences, or bizarre imagery to jog your memory. The five American Great Lakes for example can be "HOMES"—Huron Ontario Michigan Erie Superior.

• **Acronymic phrases:** these can be a good way to memorize lists and the ordering of things. For instance, to remember the planets in our solar system, you might use the following: My (Mercury) Very (Venus) Educated (Earth) Mother (Mars) Just (Jupiter) Served (Saturn) Us (Uranus) Noodles (Neptune).

→ Memory testers

Try the following exercises. Notice how much you rely on your visual memory to answer the questions.

1. This is your life

The following questions will test your long-term memory. Answer as many as you can.

A: What did you have for breakfast this morning?

B: Where were you last Sunday afternoon?

C: Where were you at midnight last New Year's Eve?

D: How did you celebrate your 21st birthday?

E: What was the last movie you saw?

F: Where were you when Barack Obama was declared President of the USA?

2. Attention to detail

Most of us are familiar with the enigmatic smile of the Mona Lisa but can you answer the following:

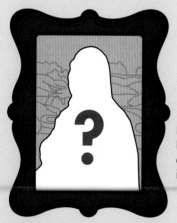

A: What color are her eyebrows?

B: In the pose, does her right hand rest on her left hand or is it left over right?

Solutions on p.173 »»

Photographic memory

Photographic, or eidetic, memory is a specific phenomenon in which people can remember perfectly anything they have seen. This memory usually fades, but it can be so accurate as to enable somebody, after seeing a picture of 1,000 randomly sprayed dots on a white sheet, to reproduce them perfectly.

For instance, a journalist called Shereshevsky noted that he could remember innumerable words and long number sequences after seeing them for only a few seconds. His memory appeared to be photographic and perfect. He could recall great chunks of information forwards or backwards even after a gap of 15 years. He used all his senses, as well as association and other mnemonic techniques to make the information he received meaningful.

But it came at a price! Shereshevsky found it hard to hold down conversations and perform other tasks that required him to use his fluid intelligence, because the information in his photographic memory set off an uncontrollable train of distracting associations.

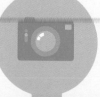

3. Number recall

Study the numbers below for 1 minute and then cover them up. Try to use ordering technique (see p.33) to organize the information. How many numbers can you recall?

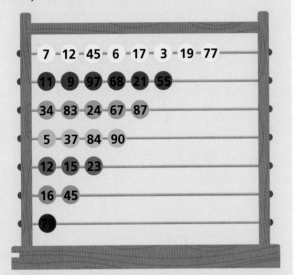

How to never forget a face

Why do we forget someone's name immediately after being introduced to them? Think about it: "this is Nina Dawes." Taken in isolation these words are meaningless. In addition, the name has no real "connection" to the face. For instance, if a person's name was Mr. Buckteeth and he had large teeth, then it would be easy to remember. In times gone by, names were based on memory and association: the man banging the anvil for your horse shoe was Mr. Blacksmith and the man selling you the leg of lamb was Mr. Butcher. Today you have to recreate that image and association to store the name. So here are few tips to help you remember:

• *On introduction ask them to repeat the name*

• *Repeat the name out loud yourself since repetition increases memory capability*

• *Study the name and form an association. In our example, you could associate the first name "Nina" to the sound an ambulance makes and link the surname to the classic rock group The Doors, to help you remember it.*

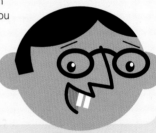

4. Spot the changes

Study the picture on the left for 1 minute. Then cover it up and circle the 6 alterations made to the same picture on the right.

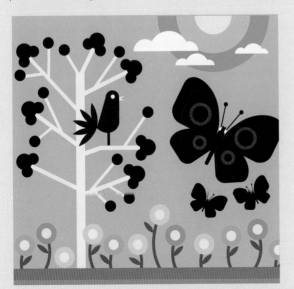

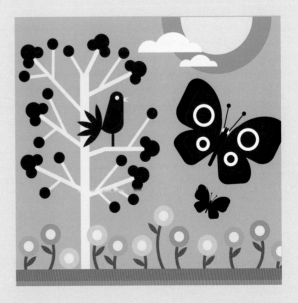

The Journey Method

The Journey Method or Method of Loci (to use its original name) is a technique for memorizing long lists of items. It has been practiced since the ancient Greek era, a time when long speeches had to be recited without recourse to notes because paper was such a luxury.

The method is a type of mnemonic link system based on memorizing items along an imagined journey or series of locations (loci) that are familiar to you. You do this by associating the object with a point in the imagined location or journey. Since the human brain thinks more readily in pictures, it is able to recall a disparate list of items a lot easier than if the information was memorized by rote, for instance.

How does it work?

Start by plotting out an imaginary journey with landmark points along the route. Do bear in mind that you will need to have visualized the journey beforehand to use this technique effectively. The landmarks (points of reference) have to be crystal clear before you hook any information on them. The characteristics of the images you choose are very important for the technique to work. They should be unusual, vivid, striking, surreal, incongruous. The goal is to make a memorable picture.

The diagram opposite is an example of a route. We have dotted items from the to do list at key points along a stroll that starts outside a house. We pass a park bench, a pond, a large tree, a school, a flower stall, a bridge, and finally a fountain. These form the key "landmark" points, which are immutable, although others can be added as you become familiar with the route. The list items have then been associated with a subject, an activity, or an object at the key points. For instance, the man on the park bench with the stethoscope is the mental trigger to book a doctor's appointment, a duck sporting a mohican relates to the hair appointment, and so on.

Why not conceive your own journey and see how many items you can recall from your own list of things to do?

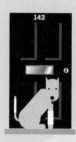

1 Front door: a bandaged dog sits on the front doorstep

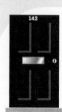

START YOUR MEMORY JOURNEY HERE

8 The fountain is spraying out letters

7 A sailing boat passes under bridge, sail stitched from items of clothing

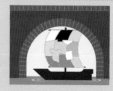

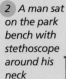
2 *A man sat on the park bench with stethoscope around his neck*
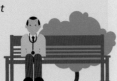

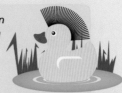
3 *The pond in the park has a duck with a bright mohawk haircut.*

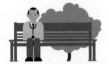
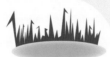

4 *A tree in the park has been struck by lightning*

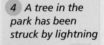
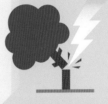

TO DO LIST

1 Give dog medicine
2 Book doctor's appointment
3 Go to hair appointment
4 Pay electricity bill
5 Buy milk
6 Buy birthday card for Mom
7 Hang out washing
8 Mail letter

5 *A teacher outside the school is drawing a cow on the blackboard*

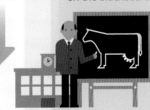

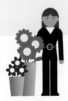

6 *The woman at the flower stall is wearing a birthday cake hat*

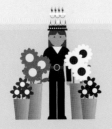

Mega memory

Memory experts believe that by applying the Journey Method a person with ordinary memorization capabilities, after establishing the route stop-points of their own "Journey," can use it to remember the sequence of a shuffled deck of cards with less than an hour of practice.

→ Expanding visual memory

5. Memory connections

Study the list of words below for 2 minutes and try to memorize as many as you can: see if you can use the Journey Method to commit the words to memory. Then cover up the list.

Book	Hand	And
White	Work	Time
If	Candle	Hold

A: Now, on a blank piece of paper, write down as many of the words as you can, and in the right order.

Visual memory

How did you find that exercise? Were some words easier to memorize than others? You might have found that it was harder to remember words that were not nouns because they were more abstract and did not lend themselves to a visual translation. We are able to place in our visual memory information such as objects, places, animals, or people, and access them more readily. A simple exercise such as this proves how effective our visual memory is. Some psychologists refer to it as the "mind's eye." Try the exercises on the next page, which incorporate a visual element, and see how you do.

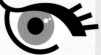

B: Can you remember the first two words of column 1?

C: Can you recall the exact central word spatially?

D: Can you remember the last word in the first column?

E: Can you remember the last word in the second column?

F: Were any words repeated?

G: Can you remember the first word in the last column?

H: What is the longest word?

6. Can you remember?

Study the pictures below for 2 minutes and then cover them up. Try to memorize as many as you can using the Journey Method (see p.36).

A: Can you remember the first three images of column 1?

B: Can you remember the central image?

C: Can you remember the last image?

D: How many animals do you remember seeing?

E: Were any images repeated?

7. Sporting chance

Allow yourself 1 minute to memorize the athletes, then cover up the pictures. Now answer the questions.

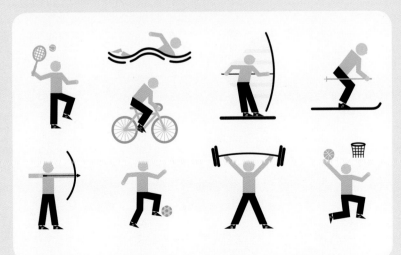

A: Are the athletes facing left or right or both directions?

B: How many sports shown involve water?

C: What is directly above the basketball player?

D: How many athletes are using equipment?

→ Pegging

Pegging is a slightly different technique from the Journey Method. The link system of the Journey Method works brilliantly for some people but not as well for others. The problem for some can be that if they forget a point in the journey they break the chain link, lose their cue, and it is hard to continue. This doesn't occur with Pegging. Pegs, like those in a cloakroom with coats and hats hung on them, have information hung on them, and they are independent of each other.

A preference for pegs

The benefit of pegs is that they provide an unmovable, stable support for whatever you are trying to memorize. A peg can be anything that you already know well and to which you can link new information. These pegs are known as loci—a location where you can mentally position a piece of information you need to recall later.

Pegging pi (π)

Let's say you had to remember the number 31 41 59 26 53 (the first 10 digits of pi (π), but it could equally be a phone number or items on a list). Your first five loci could be things in your garden: Gate, Lawn, Path, Washing line, and Tree. You then convert the numbers into other concepts using another memory technique: association. For instance, outside the gate you could have a bird (rotated "3") landing on a perch "1." The garden could have "4" children playing with a toy shaped like the number one (1), and so on and so forth.

This may sound ridiculous but with five strange but memorable images you have learned pi to 10 decimal places. In our illustrated example, the pegs are parts of the body (something you're unlikely to forget) but they could be objects within the rooms of a house (or just the rooms themselves).

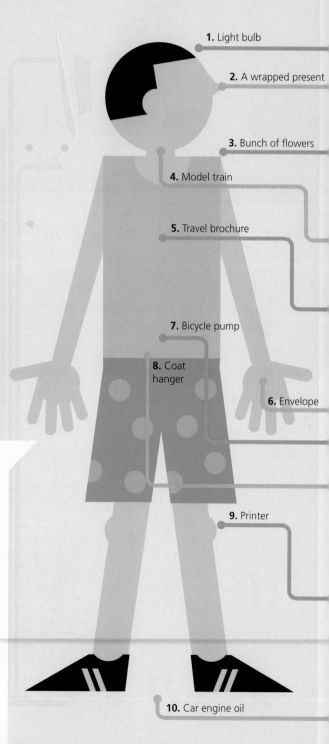

1. Light bulb
2. A wrapped present
3. Bunch of flowers
4. Model train
5. Travel brochure
7. Bicycle pump
8. Coat hanger
6. Envelope
9. Printer
10. Car engine oil

SHOPPING LIST

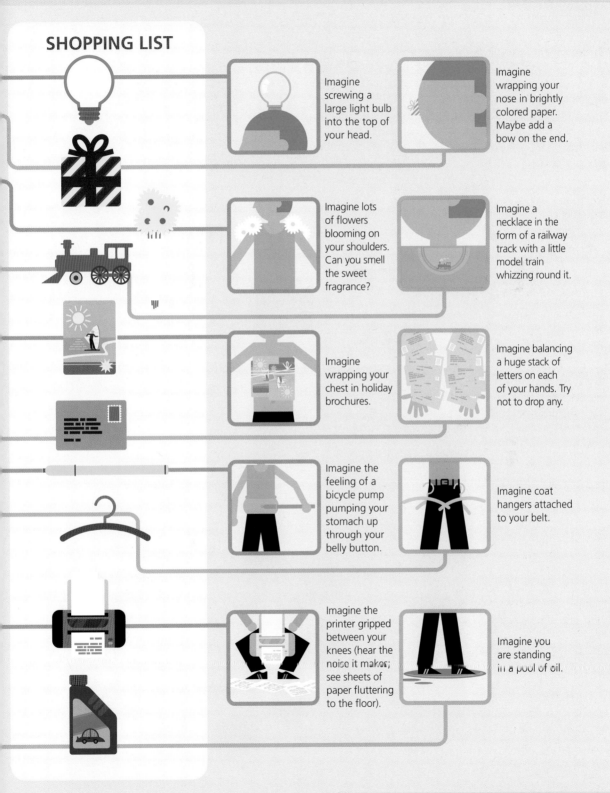

Imagine screwing a large light bulb into the top of your head.

Imagine wrapping your nose in brightly colored paper. Maybe add a bow on the end.

Imagine lots of flowers blooming on your shoulders. Can you smell the sweet fragrance?

Imagine a necklace in the form of a railway track with a little model train whizzing round it.

Imagine wrapping your chest in holiday brochures.

Imagine balancing a huge stack of letters on each of your hands. Try not to drop any.

Imagine the feeling of a bicycle pump pumping your stomach up through your belly button.

Imagine coat hangers attached to your belt.

Imagine the printer gripped between your knees (hear the noise it makes; see sheets of paper fluttering to the floor).

Imagine you are standing in a pool of oil.

→ More memory games

8. Peg that memory

Look at the illustrations below for one minute and try to memorize the items. Then cover up the pictures and recall as many as you can. Try to use the Pegging technique (see p.40) by imagining the items dotted around in your favorite room.

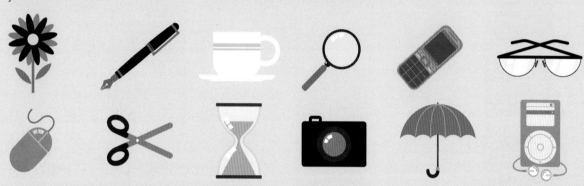

9. Noble tastes

The Knights of the Round Table are talking about their favorite vegetables. Study the diagram opposite for 2 minutes and then cover it up. Try to use an acronymic phrase to remember the knights (see p.33 for more information on acronymic phrases).

A: How many knights are present?

B: What is Sir Lucan's favorite veg?

C: Whose favorite is cabbage?

D: Who is sitting to the right of the person whose favorite vegetable is cauliflower?

E: Which two knights have names beginning with D?

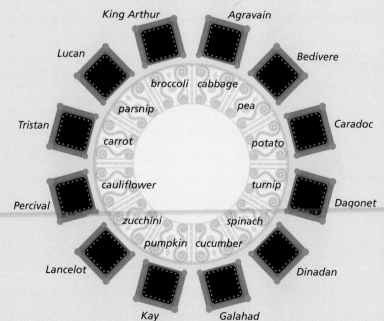

10. A sizable matter

Below is a list of random objects. Study the list for 1 minute and then cover it up. Try to use the ordering technique (see p.33) and recall them in terms of size, starting with the smallest.

Skyscraper
Dinosaur
Bus
Coffee mug
Human being
Laptop computer
Helicopter

11. Where was that?

Memorize the positioning of the arrows on the 4 x 4 grid below for 20 seconds, then cover up the diagram.

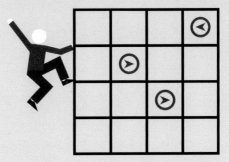

Assuming the grid runs from 1–16, left to right, horizontally, where are the arrows placed?

A: 3, 6, 9   **B:** 4, 6, 11   **C:** 5, 10, 12

12. Evocative senses

Engaging the other senses besides sight, study the images below for 1 minute and try to memorize them. If it is a food item, recall how it tastes; if it is a musical instrument, remember the sound it makes. Now cover up the images and see how many you can recall.

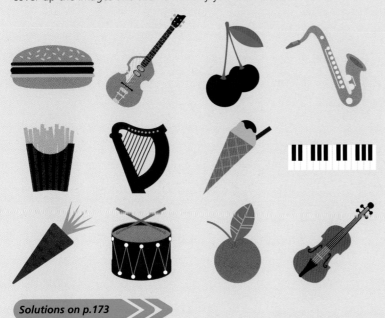

Solutions on p.173 >>>

Memory and smell

Smell is a highly effective prompt to tap forgotten memories. Have you ever caught a whiff of wood fire or a perfume and found yourself transported to a time in your past completely out of the blue, or even remembered an old lover?

Scientists believe that there is a cortex close to the limbic system that started out as a "smell brain" and evolved into an "emotional brain," which is important for memory. It is called the rhinal cortex. Therefore, the connection between smell, emotion, and memory has an anatomical basis.

Smell-evoked memories might seem clearer or more intense than other memories because they appear to be more "emotional" than memories triggered by visual, audio, or other types of cues. Studies suggest that while smells evoke memories that may feel more powerful, they don't help people recall more information, or specific details.

13. Sewing patterns

Take 1 minute to memorize the pattern on each grid
below. Then try to recreate it on the grid provided.
How many strokes can you remember accurately?

A:

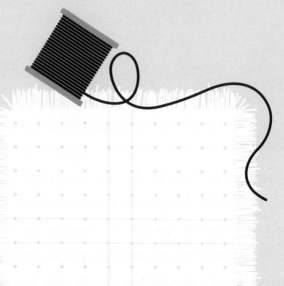

strokes

B:

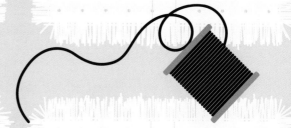

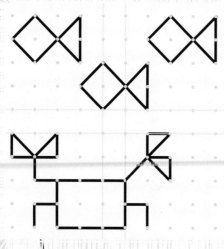

strokes

14. Memory math

The numbers have been replaced by the symbols below. Study the symbols and then cover them up and attempt the sums, trying to remember what number each symbol represents. Use an association technique (see p.33) to connect each symbol to its corresponding number.

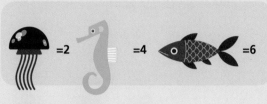

A: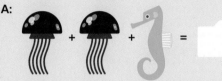

B: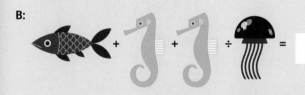

C: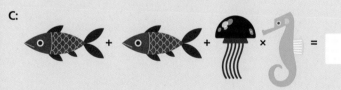

16. DIY dilemma

You're off to the hardware store to buy a few essentials but have no means to write a shopping list. Spend 2 minutes memorizing the items below, then cover up the list and see how many you can recall using the Journey Method (see p.36).

- Can of paint
- Ladder
- Ceramic tiles
- Light bulb
- Gloves
- Safety goggles
- Package of screws
- Hard hat
- Sandpaper
- Drop cloth

Solutions on p.173

15. Olympic colors

What colors make up the rings of the Olympic Games' logo? We've colored 2 rings to jog your memory.

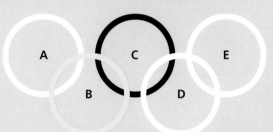

Color **A:**   Color **D:**   Color **E:**

Dreams: the perfect memory?

Sometimes we have vivid dreams of acquaintances, friends, family, and lovers we have not seen or even thought about for many years, even decades. In these dreams, however, the images we see of them are perfectly clear—all colors and details are exactly as they were in real life. This confirms that the brain is capable of tapping into memories where the images are perfect and unclouded by the passing of time. It is possible that these can be recalled with the right trigger. However, until scientists discover a way to harness this innate ability, the techniques demonstrated throughout this chapter are the most effective for organizing information so that you can accurately retrieve it at any time.

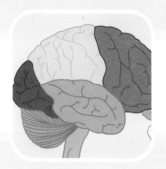 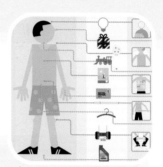

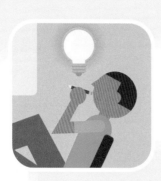 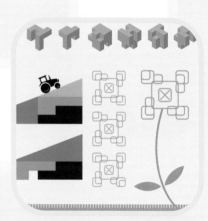

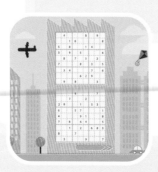 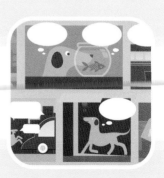

Chapter 3
Visual reasoning and spatial awareness

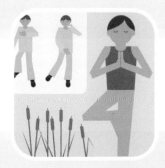

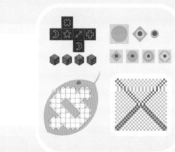

Thinking in pictures

Just consider the work your brain does when you walk to the local store to pick up a grocery item. Every step you take, you have to use 3-D visualization to navigate the space to make sure you don't bump into other people or objects. The task becomes even more complicated when you're driving a car. Things move faster and you have to use predictive vision to determine where all the other road users might be at any given moment.

You use visual and spatial reasoning within days of being born. Your visual cortex begins to adapt to light right after birth and, within weeks, you're able to separate your parents' faces from the myriad colors and shapes around you. At this stage, nothing fascinates you more than your mother's face. Then, as you grow older, you play many games to develop your visual sense. For example, when you are trying to complete a jigsaw puzzle you have to figure out how to put the pieces together to recreate the picture on the front of the box. The way the different shapes fit together hones your ability to reason, deduce, analyze, and solve problems.

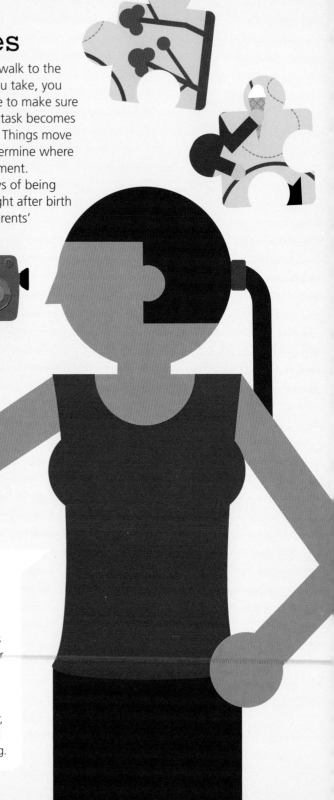

Spatial awareness

Visual and spatial thinking is, of course, important in memory—consider how taxi drivers navigate their way through the tangle of city streets. But it's also a vital skill in many other professions. Any line of work that involves complex design and arrangement, such as architecture or urban planning, demands visual thinking. The people who work in these fields rely on their ability to present ideas diagramatically. On a much smaller scale, if you're planning a day outdoors and need to fill a picnic hamper, you will have to visualize how to fit the food, plates, and utensils into the confined space before you begin loading.

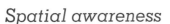

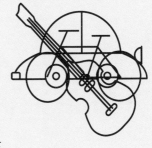

Recognition factor

Some people are blessed with these skills, others need to put more effort into sharpening that area of their brain. But there are ways in which visual and spatial intelligence can be developed. The first thing the brain has to do with visual information is recognize it.

1. Overlapped objects

Below are pictures of three objects overlapping each other. Can you figure out what each of the images are?

A:

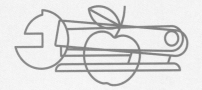

Objects:

1   2   3

B:

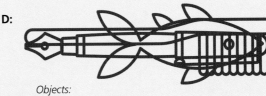

Objects:

1   2   3

C:

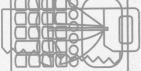

Objects:

1   2   3

D:

Objects:

1   2   3

A camel's head?

Does the shape on the right mean anything to you? Could it be a camel's head, or the head of another animal? If you recognized Africa tilted 90 degrees counterclockwise, congratulations—you're in a minority. But if you didn't, don't worry—not many people instantly identify shapes that have been tilted away from their normal axis.

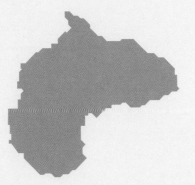

Solutions on p.174 ≫≫

Food trail

In ancient times visual intelligence used to be much more important to survival than verbal intelligence. For instance, the ability to deduce that animal footprints might lead to food is a human trait that developed during that time.

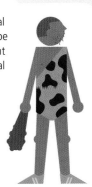

→ Seeing is learning

In contrast to other types of reasoning—such as numerical and verbal reasoning—visual reasoning is not something directly addressed in most education systems. This may be because it is already used in a variety of subjects, such as art, sports, math, and music, so perhaps there seems little point in isolating it, as you would do with verbal reasoning (languages) or numerical reasoning (math), to develop that particular mental faculty. As a result, most people never learn how to realize their full visual thinking potential. What's more, some psychologists suggest that the education system is at fault for labeling many visually gifted children as deficient because they do not fit into a verbally geared education system.

Enrich your spatial intelligence

Although your spatial reasoning skills are called upon all the time, it is usually for tasks that you do repeatedly, such as wheeling the shopping cart through the aisles of the supermarket or performing a parallel park on the familiar space of your driveway, and you tend to operate on autopilot.

In doing so, you rely on your spatial memory rather than stimulate your spatial intelligence to tackle new spaces, shapes, forms, and dimensions. A simple and efficient way to improve your spatial intelligence is by doing a 3-D mechanical puzzle, such as Rubik's cube. In addition, research has shown that playing video games has a marked effect on overall spatial awareness (see p.55). For those of you who aren't big on shoot 'em ups and racecar simulations, there are other simple ways to sharpen your spatial aptitude; see "Tips" opposite.

Benefits of visual thinking

• **Visual thinking** is a proven method of organizing ideas and finding coherent solutions to problems.

• **Visual thinking** techniques improve memory, focus, organization, critical thinking, and problem solving.

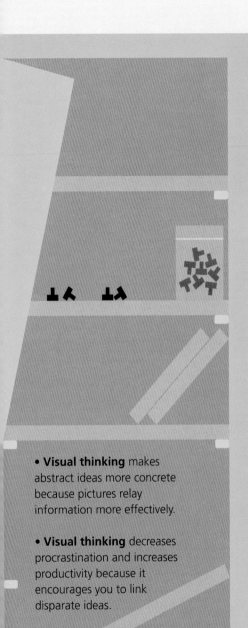

• **Visual thinking** makes abstract ideas more concrete because pictures relay information more effectively.

• **Visual thinking** decreases procrastination and increases productivity because it encourages you to link disparate ideas.

Tips

• Close your eyes and perform mental rotation of familiar things that surround you, such as the house you live in, the building where you work, or even landmarks that you might walk past every day.

• Take a class in sculpture, pottery, carpentry, or even computer design—anything that involves either calculating or manipulating things in 3-D.

• Look around you and estimate the length of objects near and far. You can do this anywhere you happen to be. Then get closer and gauge the accuracy of your estimates.

• Assemble furniture. By following the instructions on a diagram, you will develop your visual recognition skills.

• Keep doing a variety of challenging visual puzzles. (See pp.52–55 and pp.58–60.)

Depth perception

Depth perception is the ability to see the world in 3-D. We use three methods to determine depth and distance. If we have a memory of the size of an object, then the brain can gauge the distance based on the size of the object on the retina. Secondly, when we move our head from side to side, objects that are nearby move rapidly across the retina while movement of distant objects is minimal. Our brain uses this information to estimate distance. Lastly, each eye receives a slightly different image of an object, especially when an object is close to our eyes. The brain then combines this information to calculate distance.

→ Visual teasers

The following puzzles have been designed to exercise your skills of image and pattern recognition. There are others that will hone your concentration and test your logical aptitude.

2. Guess the picture

What would you see in the picture if you assembled the pieces together?

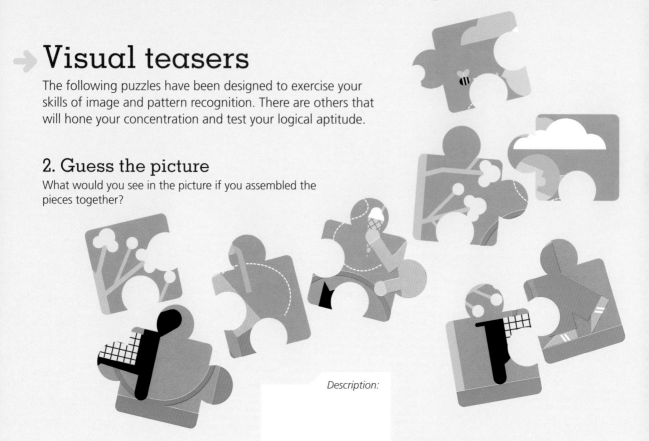

Description:

3. Triangle test

How many right-angled triangles can you create in this figure by connecting any 3 dots?

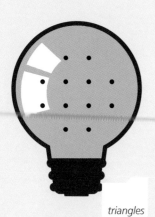

triangles

4. Spot the flipper

Take a look at the three shapes. Each one is exactly the same but one has been flipped over so that you can see the other side. For each question work out which shape has been flipped.

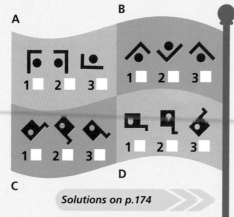

Solutions on p.174 >>

5. Cake for eight

How do you cut a cake into 8 equal-sized pieces with only 3 cuts?

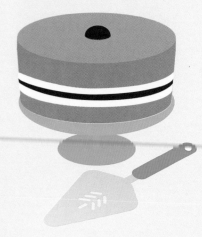

6. Reversed digits

Circle the numbers below that have
been reversed.

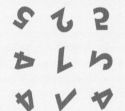

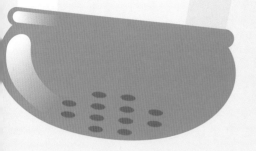

7. Quick-speed counting

A: Count the number of times the number
"6" appears below.

B: At the same time, count the number of
times both "3"s and "7"s appear in the
sequence below (don't just count all the
"3"s, and then the "7"s).

"3"s:

"7"s:

1234467889974674657865876576576

3576573625432657346578436578342

2732188582735827456724687343828

7672878682768723682376783768267

264764882317834643276487 6774653

7436574386581483627868653873456

8. Largest circle

If the circles represented by arcs
A, B, and C were completed, which
would have the greatest diameter?

A

B

C

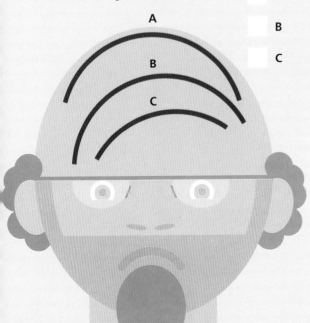

Mozart effect: does it work?

So does listening to certain types of classical music
increase spatial reasoning and improve visual
recognition? The "Mozart effect" was first mooted
in the field of childhood development in the early
1990s. The term comes from a study that claimed that
since neurons firing in specific patterns can lead to an
increase in intelligence, music could be used to activate
those patterns because the brain responds to specific
sound frequencies. The researchers conducting the study
maintained that when children receive musical stimulus
their brains form connections between neurons in
patterns that also help them with spatial reasoning.
However, a number of followup studies have found no
such correlation. In fact, many cynics believe that the
media has exaggerated and distorted the claims.

9. Straight or crooked?

Is the line across the corner of the cube straight or crooked?

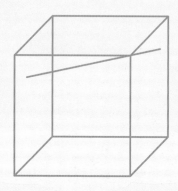

Straight: *Crooked:*

10. Phony image

Which 2 of the 6 cropped images do not belong to the picture below?

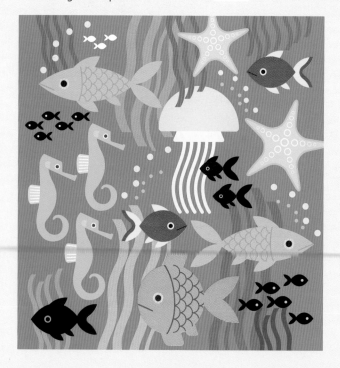

11. Largest parcel?

Assuming that the shapes below are 2-D, which of them has the largest surface area?

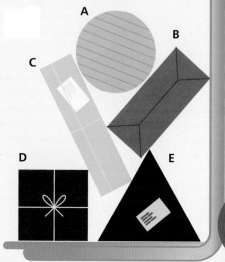

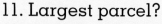

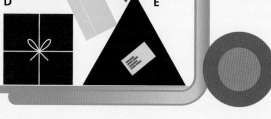

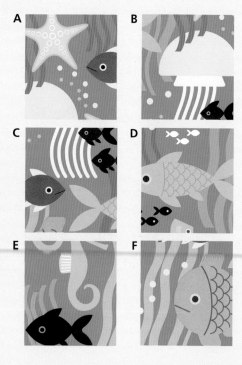

12. Sharp fox

How many triangles can you count in the picture of the fox?

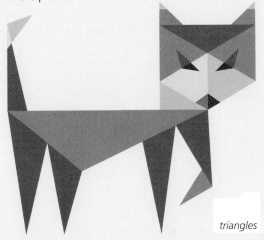

triangles

13. Counting stars

Study these overlapping stars and then answer the questions below.

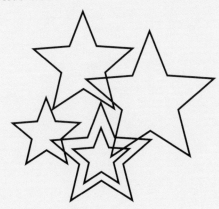

A: How many stars can you see?

B: How many triangles can you count?

C: How many stars does the largest star overlap?

Solutions on p.174

14. Solitary snowflake

All of these snowflakes appear twice except for one. Circle the snowflake that only appears once.

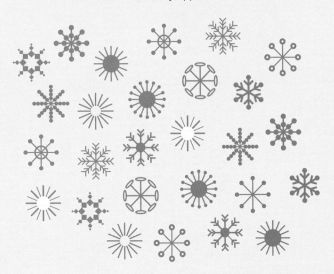

Video games

Video games are excellent for developing visual awareness. For example, recent studies show that they can significantly improve a surgeon's dexterity when performing operations. Also, playing video games has been shown to increase short-term memory of subjects in test groups. The reason for this is that most games require players to distribute their attention across the screen quickly in order to detect and react to changing events. In fact, playing video games may trigger previously inactive genes that are crucial for developing neural pathways necessary for spatial attention. Research is now suggesting that playing video games could even increase attention spans rather than reduce them.

Reading maps

Map-reading tests your spatial reasoning skills. It's a step up from simple visual recognition because not only do you have to identify symbols on a 2-D surface but you also have to relate that information to the physical space the map is referring to. It's a skill that combines reading, mental rotation, and mathematics to improve your overall spatial awareness.

When you're reading a map the right hemisphere of your brain is activated to help you stay oriented and navigate space. Studies have shown that map-reading can increase the size of the hippocampus—a key area of the brain that is responsible for spatial memory (see p.14). It is no surprise then that the size of the hippocampus in taxi drivers is generally larger, and that size actually varies according to the time they have spent in the job.

More crucially, these studies suggest that you can develop your spatial reasoning skills. Even if you consider yourself inept when it comes to reading maps, it is a skill you can master with practice. If you work hard at developing your map-reading skill, in time you'll be able to relate map symbols to terrain quickly, as well as identify key information from the map to maneuver through unfamiliar surroundings. Equally, if you rely too much on satellite navigation systems, your hippocampus will not be activated and your spatial memory will not have a reason to develop.

Shark Island

The Caves

Palm Beach

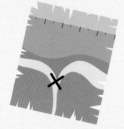 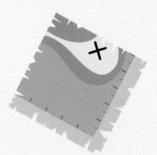

15. Find the treasure

This is a fun game to test your map-reading ability. The picture you see is of a treasure island. A treasure chest is buried somewhere on it. A map showing its location has been cut into nine pieces, which are randomly distributed over the page. "X" marks the position of each of the nine landmarks on the island, and the location of the treasure is marked with a coin.

Your aim is to mentally assemble the pieces by squaring each piece with the picture and drawing it into the grid. You'll then be able to identify the square where the treasure is located.

A	B	C
D	E	F
G	H	I

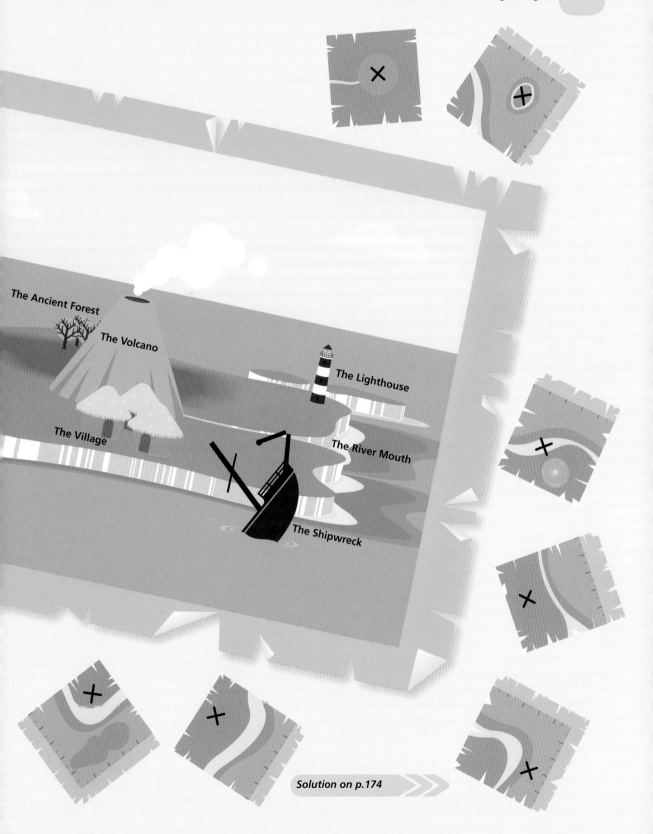

The Ancient Forest

The Volcano

The Lighthouse

The Village

The River Mouth

The Shipwreck

Solution on p.174

Mental rotation puzzles

The following puzzles and exercises are slightly more difficult. They will not only test your visual recognition skills but also your ability to accurately visualize objects in 3-D and perform mental rotation.

16. Origami enigma

If you fold the image along the dotted line, which shape would you see?

17. Shape shifting

If you rotate this shape 90° in a clockwise direction, which of the four shapes would you see?

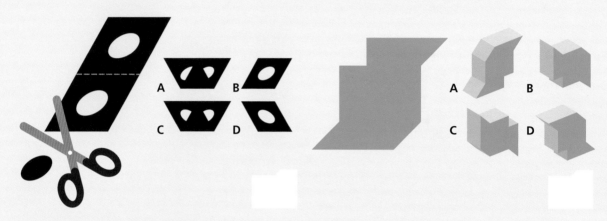

18. Stacking mosaic tiles

If you placed these tiles on top of each other, starting with the largest at the bottom, which image would you see?

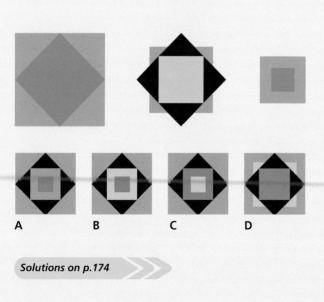

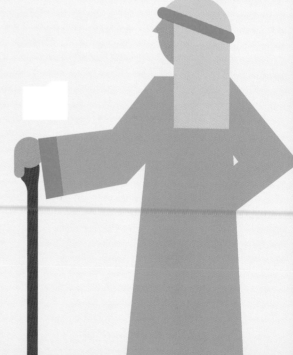

Solutions on p.174

19. Squaring up

These shapes have been cut out of a square. However, an extra shape has been added to the assortment. Can you identify the rogue shape?

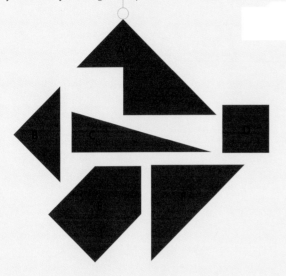

21. False pattern

Look at the pattern on this teacup. Now look at the four options below—which of them does not have the same pattern?

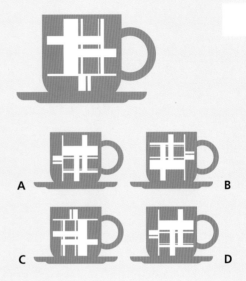

20. The correct cube

If you folded the template into a cube, which of the four options underneath might you see?

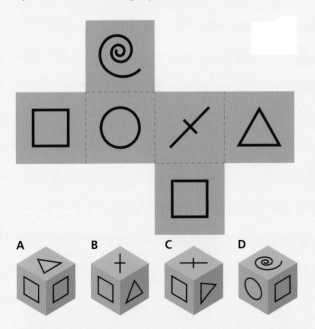

Men and women

There are subtle differences in the way men and women mentally visualize objects in 3-D. Scientists have discovered that there is a region in the cerebral cortex called the inferior parietal lobule that is responsible for processing spatial information and is generally larger in men than in women. Does this mean that women have poor spatial awareness? Not at all. Many women are fantastic at math and physics. Only when you analyze large populations for slight but significant trends do you see any difference.

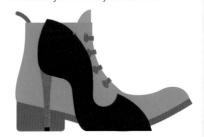

22. Perfect fit

Identify the correct piece from the selection below that completes the cube.

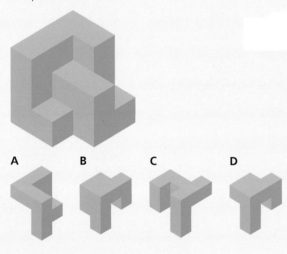

23. On a roll

If you rotate this shape 90° in a clockwise direction, which of the four shapes will you see?

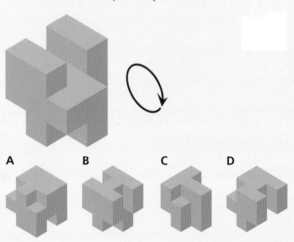

24. The vanishing area

When the same pieces are rearranged to form the second triangle, a gap emerges. Can you explain the change in the size of the surface area?

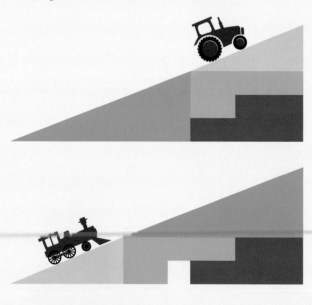

25. Spinning blossom

When rotated 180° in a clockwise direction, what does the flower head look like?

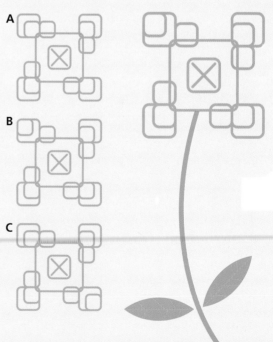

Visual thinking and the imagination

Don't think of a pink elephant. You couldn't help it, could you? Our guess is that you've just pictured a pink elephant. This is a simple experiment to prove two things: one, that imagination is synonymous with the mind's eye, and two, we are all blessed with the ability to visualize beyond what is real. Creative thinkers, such as painters and filmmakers, rely on their ability to generate concepts in the visual form. They cast their mind's eye into the vast sea of endless possibilities and try to search for original solutions to old problems. This ability to visualize allows them to transcend traditional ideas and ingrained conventions

to create meaningful new ideas and methods. The practice of visual thinking to solve problems, work through issues, and communicate clearly has been fundamental to human progress in every civilization. You don't have to be an artist to think visually. It's all about paying closer attention to your inner eye, seeing beyond the obvious, and entertaining brand new ideas.

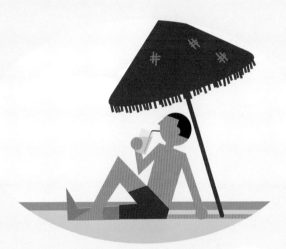

Capture the daydream

Next time you catch yourself daydreaming, try to grab the moment by writing down the details. You'll find that you're describing a series of images. Or, if you can, keep a pen and some paper by your bed and, as soon as you wake up, note down what you can remember of your dreams. You might find yourself describing a set of surreal pictures that make no logical sense.

What you will have done is echo the beginnings of the creative process. It is an example of the kind of visual thinking that people working in creative industries often do. You too can get the most out of your imagination. Refer to Chapter 4 to learn ways of boosting your creative thinking.

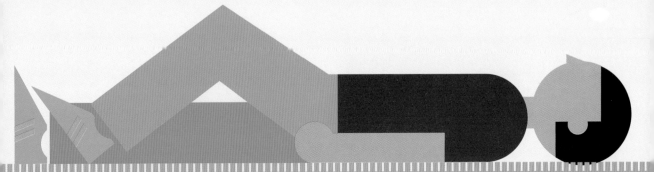

Mind Maps

A Mind Map is a useful visual tool for exploring and examining an idea, a task, or a problem. Invented by psychology author Tony Buzan, it is a diagram that you produce by writing down all the elements of the given problem, which branch out from a central key word or idea. The aim is to organize disparate thoughts into a coherent whole.

The benefits of Mind Maps

Mind Maps offer flexibility of thought, since you are visualizing a problem in a radial, graphical, and nonlinear manner. They also call on your logical and creative skills, thereby demanding work from both sides of your brain. In addition, a Mind Map allows you to see the whole picture at once on a single page. You'll find that your brain has a natural inclination to look for patterns and completion.

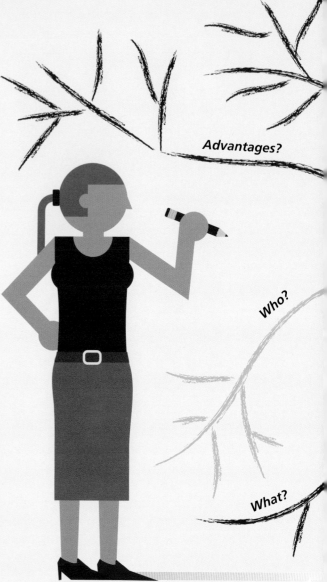

How does it work?

The elements are arranged instinctively, according to what you consider important, and these sprawl out on the page via curved branches. A typical Mind Map starts with a single word or idea placed in the center, to which associated ideas are added. Although you take a brainstorming approach, you place all the ideas into specific groups. You can use different colors to separate these groups.

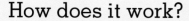

Most Mind Maps have three crucial parts:
• A central word or image—the subject
• Branches reaching out in all directions from the subject—main themes
• Less important themes— branches or offshoots that carry collateral information

An example

Philippa is considering a career change. She is thinking about leaving the field of IT to become a journalist but remains uncertain. She draws a Mind Map to help her make the right choice. Her central question is: Do I want to be a journalist? Then she begins with several primary questions: Why do I want to be journalist? How can I make it happen? Where can I pursue this career? When can I do this? What do I need to use? Who can help me? What advantages might the career have?

Disadvantages?

Why?

How?

Where?

When?

Association: think of everything you can associate with any of the headings and write them down along the branches. You'll find you start thinking of some related ideas. Start a sub-branch where you think it fits best and put down all these ideas as well. You might want to use a different colored pen for the new branch. Soon, you will find your brain trying to make connections between all the ideas you write down.

Analysis: look at what you've drawn. Which branches contain more information? Where are the uncertainties? Use the diagram to reflect on your thoughts. This may lead you to start another Mind Map.

Whatever action you decide to take, the process of Mind Mapping will have helped you generate and crystallize your ideas. There are two further stages to undergo before you master the technique: **Application** (continued practice) and **Adaptation** (personalizing the tool to suit your needs). If you begin to use Mind Maps on a frequent basis, you will soon find that there are no limitations to the variety of ways you can use the model, since there are no limits to the number of connections that your brain can make. For further information you can visit www. buzanworld.com

The five "A"s

The initial principle of Mind Mapping involves following the instructions of three of the five **"A"s**: **Acceptance**, **Association**, and **Analysis**.

Acceptance: when you start a Mind Map you should set aside any preconceptions about your own limitations, and look objectively at the problem. Write down the problem or goal in the center of the page and circle it. Draw eight lines from this circle and write key headings, such as:

1. Why?
2. How?
3. Where?
4. When?

5. What (to use)?
6. Who (can help)?
7. Advantages?
8. Disadvantages?

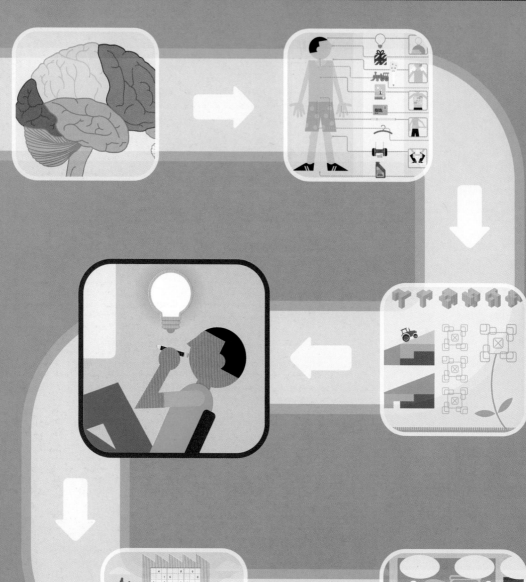

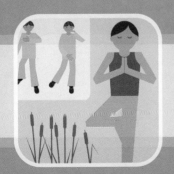

Chapter 4
Think creatively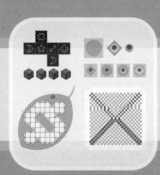

→ Demystifying creativity

So what do we mean by creativity? Fundamentally, it's a mixture of original thinking, insight, ingenuity, and innovation. Naturally, some people are born with a greater tendency to tap into their creativity (note how many times artistic and musical talent seem to run in families), but much of that results from encouragement and opportunity. A positive role model always helps. So, if for some reason you think you're not creative, perhaps it's the negative belief that is holding you back, or the lack of encouragement, rather than the level of your creative aptitude.

The creative geniuses

Where does this creative spirit come from? The images of the English Romantic poets Shelley and Byron striking a heroic pose on the rooftop in the midst of an electrical storm have seduced the world into believing that all inspiration comes like a bolt of lightning. Dramatic perhaps, but it couldn't be further from the truth. Archimedes may well have jumped out of the bath and cried "Eureka!" the instant he worked out how to calculate the volume of an irregular shaped object, but we're fairly sure that he'd visited the bathhouse fairly often before reaching that breakthrough moment. Mozart was writing symphonies at an astonishingly young age, but is he remembered for any those early compositions? Of course not, because he had to serve his apprenticeship before he could fulfill his undoubted genius. And how many unworkable theorems did Einstein devise before he thought up his Theory of Relativity? The truth of the matter is that whichever creative genius you can name, you can rest assured that his or her creation not only took a lot of brainpower, but practice and patience as well.

The cogs of creativity

Creativity is not a bolt from the blue but a process, a series of incremental steps that leads to the magic "Eureka!" moment. Social psychologist Graham Wallas produced one of the earliest models of the creative process in 1926, proposing that creative thinking goes through four distinct phases:

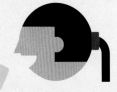

4. Verification—the final phase when the idea is worked into a form that can be proven and communicated to others.

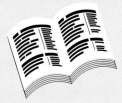

3. Illumination—the moment when a solution presents itself, albeit in a rough state.

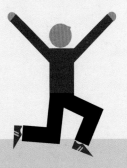

1. Preparation—the period of research, when raw material is gathered and organized, to be in a position to start the creative act.

2. Incubation—the stage when the problem is laid to one side, allowing intuition, emotion, and the unconscious mind to ponder over it.

Right-brain = creative?

As much as it is wrong to think that creative people are only those blessed with an innate genius, it is equally wrong to think that *all* creative people are naturally right-brained while all left-brained people are analytical and orderly (see p.15). The statistics might suggest that creative people tend to have a more dominant right-sided brain, but that doesn't mean that the rest of us can't be creative. The truth is everyone has the ability to be creative. In fact, creativity flourishes best when you use both sides of your brain. As proposed by Wallas' model (see above), creativity is not some magical state of mind but a series of actions that depend on logic and applied thinking as well—processes that are largely performed by the left side of the brain. What's more, brain scans have revealed that during creative thinking both hemispheres of the brain share the task equally. So, while you may have heard stories of artists feeling that they were taken over by some higher power during a creative act, the science leans more toward the theory that novel ideas materialize when imagination and analysis work side by side. Creativity is, therefore, *whole-brained* and only by integrating various mental faculties can you maximize your untapped creative potential. You can develop your ability to think creatively by learning a few popular strategies described on the following pages.

Music as a muse

This is a simple warm-up exercise to get your creative juices flowing. Listen to a piece of music without lyrics. It can be classical, jazz, dance, any type—although the slower, the better because it will help you relax. Think about the story you imagine the music is telling you. Write down the story at the end of the piece, embellish it as much as you like; don't concern yourself with form or structure.

➔ Don your creative cap

It is essential for you to be in the right state of mind to realize your full creative potential. Although this may seem to be obvious, it is something that science has been researching for a long time. For example, several years ago, neuroscientists in Australia claimed that they had found a way to "switch on" a person's unconscious creative skills by magnetic stimulation. They argued that everyone possesses extraordinary creative powers, but the problem is tapping into these reserves, for which one has to be intensely focused.

Finding focus

The ability to focus greatly determines your creativity at any given time. For example, have you never become so engrossed in an activity, such as staring at a painting, that your mind has been transported to a different time and place? Think about the last time you were curled up with an amazing novel—a real page-turner. As you became more absorbed in the story, your inner eye went into a Zen-like state, conjuring up all sorts of images of faces and places. Admittedly, you were stimulated by the quality of the writer's storytelling, but the images you fashioned were unique—each the product of your creative mind. No two people reading the same novel visualize the details in the same way, hence our occasional disappointment with

Tips

• From the previous warm-up exercise, you'll realize that music is a great stimulus. Anecdotal evidence suggests that classical music helps logical thinking, rock music helps boost energy, and dance music aids creative writing—the relentless rhythms act as a strong stimuli over a short period. Of course, these are general assertions and you will have to find for yourself what music works best for you.

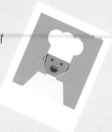

• Find a painting depicting a human figure. Concentrate on the image. Pretend you're that person: put yourself into their shoes—what do you see, how do you feel, where might you be heading, and how might you get there? Ask yourself as many questions as you can and write the answers down.

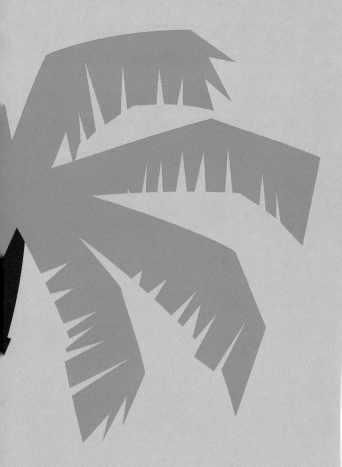

Zero in!

For those of you who are easily distracted, concentration exercises can be an effective way to enter this state. Next time you are about to start something creative, try this warm-up:

Find a quiet, comfortable place. Close your eyes and focus on your breathing first. Do not think of anything else. Take your time.

Once you feel relaxed, think of the most beautiful place you've ever been. This could be a vacation destination, such as a sun-kissed beach, the beautiful interior of a palatial building, or even the treehouse from your childhood. Use all your senses to imagine this ideal place: what do you see, what do you smell, what can you touch? Is there sand pushing between your toes, are the colors bright and dazzling, can you smell the green wilderness? Take as long as you need to picture the location in your mind. Then savor it, revel in all the minute details. Imagine walking around the area, keep searching for new elements to add to this mental composition, and focus on the new discovery. If it's an object, such as a pebble in the sand, imagine picking it up and turning it over—see all the marks on it.

Once you are immersed in the picture, you should feel totally focused. You are now in the creative spirit. Your mind's eye has been catapulted to a different time and place. Even though the location may have a basis in reality, you'll find that you have created some of the details since memory is selective (see p.30) and you've filled in the gaps by relying on your imagination. Who said you're not creative?

film adaptations. Any creative task demands your fullest attention. Somehow you must eliminate any distractions so that you can concentrate only on the task. This will establish a space in your mind where your creative spirit can roam free to be playful and inventive.

• If you're outside or near a window, stare at the clouds for five minutes and see what images your mind forms. Then use those images to write a short story.

• Alternatively, if it's night and you are lucky enough to be under a starry sky, try to see what constellations you can form. You'll be surprised at what your imagination conjures up.

→ Creative treats

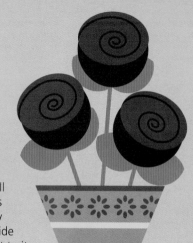

Here is a selection of great exercises to stimulate your imagination. Some you can do alone, others are group exercises, but they're all great fun and rewarding.

1. The hidden story

Spend a moment looking around the room and find the most interesting-looking object, such as a painting hanging on the wall or an ornate vase. Now imagine there is a dark secret behind this object—the sort of thing that would sit at the center of a fantasy novel. Note down a few special things that make it a secret. Decide how you would keep its secret if a master criminal was out to get to it.

That's all there is to it. By generating your own puzzling circumstances, you will have entered a more creative frame of mind. Ask yourself how C. S. Lewis came up with the idea of Narnia. Perhaps he was staring at a wardrobe?

2. Striking similes

Creative writers use similes to compare two things to create a new meaning. Often they are visually orientated and instantly make a sentence more interesting. Similes use the words "as" or "like" to make the connection between two things that are being compared. For example: "the robbers made their getaway as fast as lightning," or "the baby clung to his mother like a limpet."

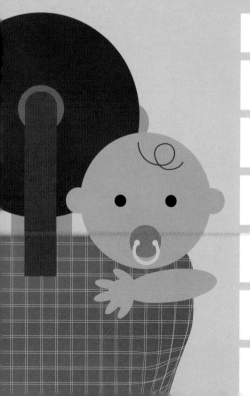

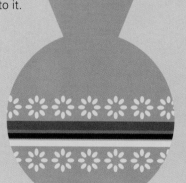

Think of a simile to complete each of the following sentences. Try to think beyond clichés and continue on a separate sheet of paper if necessary:

• Penny's smile was as sweet as……………………………………

• Johnny was a big man. He was built like………………

• The bird was as beautiful as……………………………

• The thief didn't make a sound. He moved like…………

• The sea was as calm as……………………………………

• I love a slice of cake. It's rich and sweet like…………………

• When the earthquake struck, the ground shook like…………

• She was good at playing the piano. Her fingers moved over the keys as fast as……………………………………

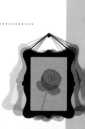

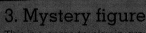

3. Mystery figure

This is a game to play in groups of four. Each of you starts with a fresh sheet of paper.

Decide on a "name" to call the figure each of you is about to draw. This is the only stimulus that binds you creatively to each other. Each person draws a head on their sheet of paper. The sheet is folded to hide the drawing and is swapped with another person in the group. During the next stage everyone draws the body, folding the sheet once again to hide the creation, and swaps it again with another person. The same is done with the legs and the feet. Once everyone is finished, unfold the drawings. You should have four completely different versions, all inspired by that name.

4. Imaginary biography

This is a game to play in groups of two or more people. Write down an assortment of words relating to fame—these could include names of celebrities, famous landmarks, or famous historical events. Put all the words into a hat. Each person takes a turn to talk about their own life for one minute. At the 30-second mark, the person reaches into the hat and picks out a word at random. Whatever the word, the person has to include it in their biography for the next 30 seconds.

Passion and purpose

Weren't these exercises a lot of fun? When was the last time you gave your imagination free licence in this way? You may not be used to thinking creatively in your day-to-day life, in which case you are neglecting a key mental faculty. One of the most ardent advocates of the belief that we are not using our creative resources properly is the Englishman Sir Kenneth Robinson.

He argues persuasively that by tapping into our creativity, we reinvigorate our passion, which breathes purpose back into our life. Robinson reminds us that the creative spirit is an essential part of human nature and human progress, and we allow our creativity to be neglected at our peril. So, if you feel that you're stuck in a rut, or you're clock-watching all day and work isn't much fun, then it might be because your creative skills are lying dormant and your brain is craving some kind of change. Perhaps it's time to find something creative to breathe passion and purpose back into your life?

→ Creative conundrums

The following puzzles are designed to get you to think creatively about a solution. This exercise isn't about finding the "right" answer because, occasionally, there might not be a definitive answer to a problem. It's about finding a solution that you think answers the problem. You may want to write your answer on a separate sheet of paper.

5. Horsing around

A man stands in the center of a field. There are 4 horses in the field, one at each corner—a bay horse, a chestnut horse, a white horse, and a black horse. The man has to tether his horses so that they can't bolt. If he must remain at the center of the field while the horses stay at the 4 corners, how can he ensure that his horses can't escape using only 3 lassos?

   If you find a solution quickly, try for another. There are at least 3 different solutions to the problem.

6. Doubling the window size

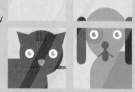

How can a square window be made twice as large without increasing its height or width? Try to think of as many solutions as possible.

7. Enough fish

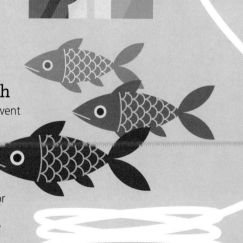

2 fathers and 2 sons went fishing one day. They spent the whole day fishing and only caught 3 fish. One father said, that is enough for all of us, we will have one each. Explain how can this be possible?

8. Drinking glasses

6 drinking glasses stand in a row, with the first 3 full of water and the next 3 empty. By handling and moving only 1 glass at a time, how can you arrange the 6 glasses so that no full glass stands next to another full glass, and no empty glass stands next to another empty glass? What do you think is the minimum number of moves required to solve this puzzle?

9. The elder twin

One day Kerry celebrated her birthday. Two days later her older twin brother, Terry, celebrated his birthday. How come?

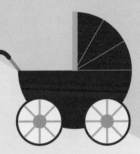

10. The swimmer in the forest

Deep in the forest, the body of a man was found wearing only swimming trunks, a snorkel, and goggles. The nearest lake was eight miles away and the sea was 100 miles away. How had he died?

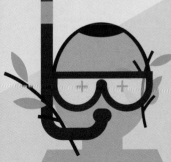

Note: this is supposedly based on a true incident.

11. Crossing the bridge

A rock band has a concert that starts in 17 minutes and its members must all cross a bridge to get there. All 4 men begin on the same side of the bridge. You must help them across to the other side. It is night. There is 1 flashlight. A maximum of 2 people can cross at one time. Any pair or individual that crosses must have the flashlight with them. The flashlight must be walked back and forth, it cannot be thrown.

Each band member walks at a different speed. A pair must walk together at the rate of the slower man's pace: **The singer:** 1 minute to cross. **The guitarist:** 2 minutes to cross. **The keyboard player:** 5 minutes to cross. **The drummer:** 10 minutes to cross. For example, if the singer and the drummer walk across first, 10 minutes have elapsed when they get to the other side of the bridge. If the drummer then returns with the flashlight, a total of 20 minutes have passed and you have failed the mission.

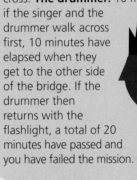

Note: there is no trick behind this. It is the simple movement of resources in the appropriate order. There are two known answers to this problem.

Solutions on p.175

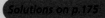

→ Surviving the creative process

Entering the creative spirit is one thing, but what happens when you're in the middle of a creative task, such as making a birthday card, a collage, or even trying some creative writing? Does your creativity come out in a continuous stream? Is the process effortless from the moment you don your creative cap? Of course not! It's not meant to be an easy process, especially if you are striving for originality. In fact, the product of any creativity emerges only after you've fought a grueling battle inside your head. You're fighting against existing modes and conventions, ideas that are ingrained and upon which your brain has successfully relied to make sense of the world around you.

Essentially, you are searching for multiple solutions rather than settling for the first idea that comes to you. Fighting against this natural inclination can be frustrating but you have to give yourself permission to be playful and inquisitive, flexible and versatile. Also, you have to remember that the creative process isn't a serene boat ride. It is more like a rollercoaster, filled with peaks and dips. For help in surviving the creative process, see our tips:

1: Acknowledge that creativity comes in cycles. You might have the seed of an idea but it is not ready to germinate. Accept that there will be periods when your creative brain might seem dormant. If you remain committed to the task, you'll find that your idea will suddenly blossom, or even shoot in an unexpected direction, and you'll reap the fruits of your commitment.

2: Embrace fear. Creativity by definition asks you to venture into uncharted territory. You're bound to make wrong turns along the way and reach dead ends. Each time, you'll be stricken by that familiar fear of failure, but reinterpret the feeling as performance energy and just keep going.

3: Shift location. If you're working on a creative task from your desk, your senses are fixed on the surroundings. This can curb your creativity so change location from time to time. Work in a different room, or go to a quiet café. Sometimes you can gain new perspective on a problem by simply shifting the direction of your chair.

4: Reconnect with your inner child. It will release you from the chains of adult sensibilities, allowing you to consider the seemingly "ridiculous" as an option. To get into this state of mind, try to delight in any childlike behavior before you begin your creative task.

5: Don't try to be perfect!
Perfection is an ideal. It's when the bar is set above and beyond your sightline. Aiming for the unattainable will only prevent you from beginning a creative task in the first place.

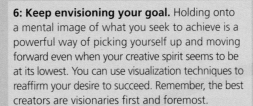

6: Keep envisioning your goal. Holding onto a mental image of what you seek to achieve is a powerful way of picking yourself up and moving forward even when your creative spirit seems to be at its lowest. You can use visualization techniques to reaffirm your desire to succeed. Remember, the best creators are visionaries first and foremost.

7: Note it down. Since your creative brain has a tendency to come up with solutions without warning, keep a small notebook and pen with you. Use them to jot down sudden brainwaves, or even an innocuous strand of an idea that might lead to a breakthrough later on. Your notepad is your net because you'll be surprised at how quickly an idea can slip through your brain.

The creative journey
Creative thinking is chaotic. Eventually, you will find a viable solution but your progress will be tumultuous. Psychologists refer to this as "loose associative thinking." It is a type of thinking that forsakes linearity for something more "jumpy." Psychologists say that the feeling of uncertainty is necessary for the human mind to be able to come up with new ideas. They claim that comfort strangles associative thinking, often leading to an answer that is timeworn or banal. Leveraging uncertainty, riding it, and valuing it are all critical to developing creative ideas.

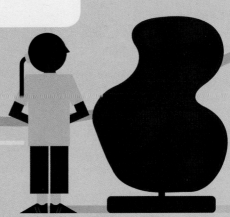

8: Visit an art gallery or museum. If you've hit a brick wall, perhaps you need a bit of space from inside your head. Galleries and museums or any other "creative place" provide superb visual stimuli to kick-start an exhausted mind. These are "play areas" where you can connect with an artist's unique take on the world. This can help release the checks you've imposed on your own creativity.

→ Doodle art

We are fairly certain that the first time you picked up a pen or a pencil you didn't write a sonnet or draw a masterpiece. You probably scribbled something that made no sense. However, encouraged by your parents and teachers, you kept doodling away and with time and practice, the squiggles developed, and found a form—probably of your house, or mom and dad, or pet dog or cat.

Doodling is one of the earliest ways in which you express your creativity. We believe that you're never too old to doodle because it can also help organize thoughts, feelings, and experiences. Like any creative endeavor, doodling can be an outlet to express what words lack, and can even offer an answer when you feel creatively trapped.

We have provided you with a set of random scribbles. All you have to do is interpret what you think each looks like—use your imagination—and begin adding to the squiggle. Draw in details or the background to flesh out your interpretation. Even if you can't think of anything, just begin adding to it until something tangible forms.

Below is an example:

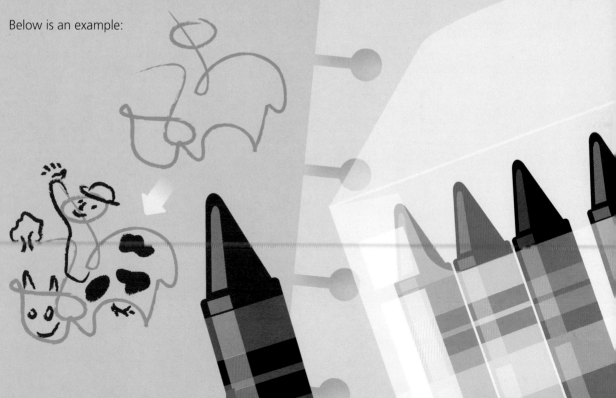

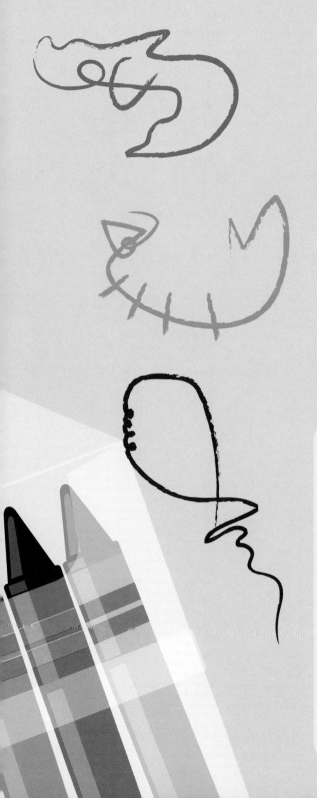

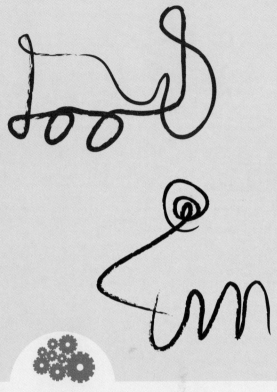

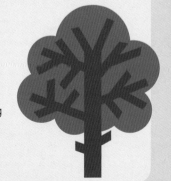

Breathing for inspiration

Has your creativity ground to a halt? Instead of letting frustration get the better of you, try to sit back and take a few deep breaths. Did you know that drawing a deep breath gives your creativity a boost by increasing the negative ions in oxygen? The negatively charged oxygen circulates throughout the brain, refreshing the neurons and, because these negative ions promote alpha waves of longer amplitude in the brain, which are associated with creative thinking, suddenly your creativity receives a recharge. So, next time your creative spirit feels deflated, spend two minutes taking deep breaths, inhaling and exhaling every five seconds, and repeat the cycle at least 12 times.

→ Thinking outside the box

You may have heard the expression "lateral thinking," which is a method of getting us to think in unorthodox ways about a problem. Psychologist Edward de Bono, who coined the phrase, believes that we tend to overuse logic and follow linear paths in our creative thinking, consequently ignoring the open spaces that flow out to the sides. In other words, "logic" then becomes counterproductive because we box ourselves in and produce the same solution to a problem, which, let's face it, isn't the least bit creative!

Lateral thinking relies on reasoning that is not immediately obvious, and encourages ideas that you may not think of by relying on logic. Lateral thinking is concerned with the perception part of thinking. It is about rewiring the way you approach a problem. De Bono describes lateral thinking with this metaphor: "You cannot dig a hole in a different place by digging the same hole deeper." Think about it. Trying harder in the same direction, especially if the direction is wrong, will not lead to any progress, and might actually hinder the chances of a breakthrough because you will only be squandering precious creative energy. Lateral thinking asks you to dig as many holes as you can. Each time you dig a new hole you uncover a new possibility. It might work or it might not. If it does, then great! If not, you simply dig another hole and continue your search.

Lateral thinking in three steps:

1. Identify the dominant ideas that prevent original ways of seeing the problem.
2. Approach the same problem from different angles, regardless of how random the angle might seem.
3. Put a stop to any doubts, preconceptions, and prejudices that might dismiss original thought.

Lateral thinking:

How many different ways are there to join all nine dots in the square using a maximum of four straight lines and without taking your pen off the paper?

HERE ARE SOME EXAMPLES

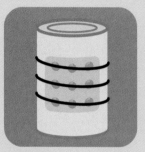

6. And if that sounds a bit far-fetched, you could do the same thing by rolling the paper into a cylinder.

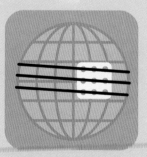

5. If you laid the paper on the ground, you could draw one long line, which circles the earth three times, joining one row of dots each time.

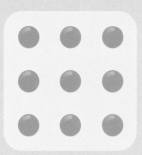

The nine dot puzzle

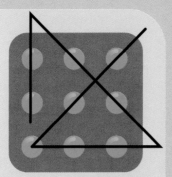

1. The standard solution: You run the pen outside the nine dot boundary to join the dots.

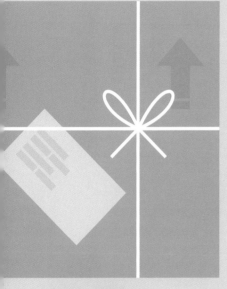

2. If you had a thick pencil, you could join the dots with just three lines.

3. Why stop at three lines? Why not take a very thick pencil and do the job with just one line?

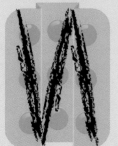

4. Even with a thinner pencil, You could still make do with three lines by folding the paper so that the dots were closer to each other.

Top tips

- **Challenge assumptions**—don't just fall back on accepted ways of thinking but question everything that has been done or is known.
- **Find focal objects**—pick an object at random (or a word from a dictionary) and see what thoughts the object or word inspires.
- **Harvest ideas**—when you've come up with as many new ideas as you can, begin the process of harvesting by selecting the best ones.
- **Invent alternatives**—allow yourself plenty of time to come up with new ideas, perhaps setting yourself a minimum (say, 50) before you begin your analysis.
- **Provide provocation**—deliberately set up a wild counterpart to the normally accepted idea, not as an end in itself, but as a possible pathway to new ideas.
- **Shape concepts**—look closely at clusters of ideas that have sprung up and see whether you can group any together into concepts.
- **Suspend judgment**—don't rush to judge any new ideas, however strange they may appear at first.

Just go crazy!

While thinking laterally, you are encouraged to consider trivial or ridiculous ideas. This is because you are using the information not for its own value but for its knock-on effect. Each idea is a stepping stone to another idea. You will probably head into many strange directions as you jump from one idea to another but at some stage you will reach an innovative solution.

→ Matchstick mayhem

Matchstick puzzles offer an excellent way to exercise your lateral thinking ability. Why spend money on expensive games when you can occupy your free time by doing these fun puzzles? The puzzles are not all solved in the same way. They require you to think outside the box and entertain myriad possibilities. The puzzles encourage you to exercise different thinking styles. You will need a box of matches or toothpicks.

12. The third square
Move 4 matches to make 3 squares.

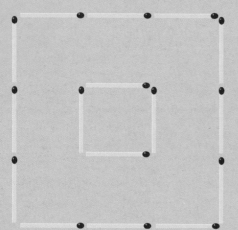

13. Three for two
Move 3 matches to make 2 squares.

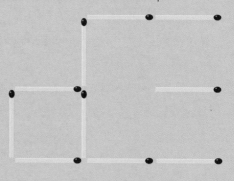

15. Swimming fish
Turn the fish by moving only 2 matches; no overlapping.

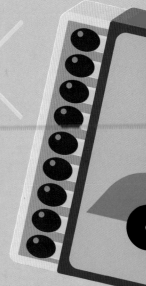

14. Remove a square
Move 2 matches to new positions to get only 4 squares, leaving no overlapping or loose ends.

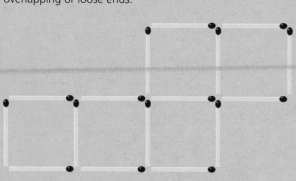

16. Try for five

Move 6 matches so that 5 squares are formed.

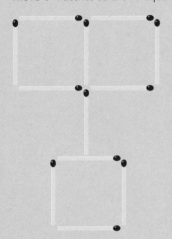

18. All the threes

Move 3 matches so that 3 squares are formed.

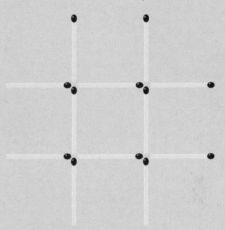

17. Even out

Move 3 matches to new positions to get only 4 squares, leaving no overlapping or loose ends.

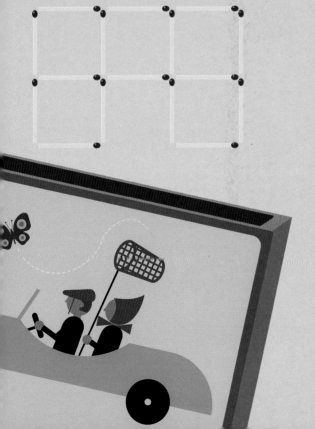

19. Total wipeout

Remove 9 matches, leaving no square (of any size), or any overlapping or loose ends.

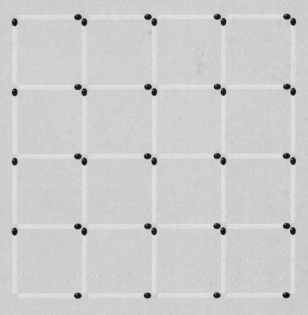

Solutions on p.176

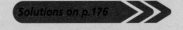

20. Equal divide

Use the 4 matches to divide the large square into 2 parts of the same shape. Use the matches without breaking or overlapping them.

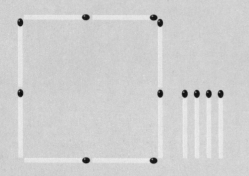

21. Find the extra triangle

Move 3 matches to make 4 equilateral triangles, without overlapping.

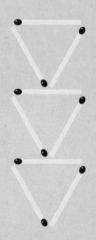

22. Break the wheel

Move 4 matches to form 3 equilateral triangles.

23. More for less

Move 3 matches to add an equilateral triangle to the square and the rhomboid.

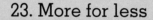

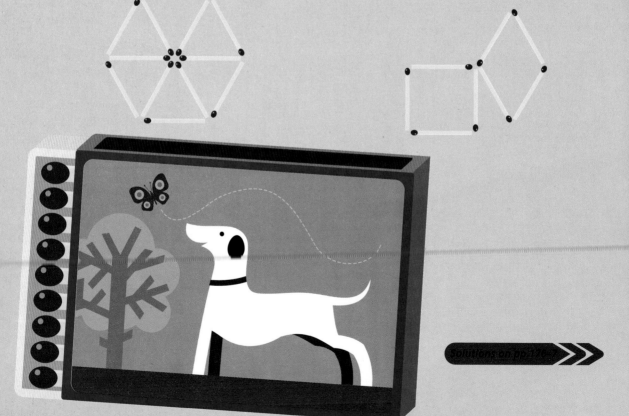

Solutions on pp.126–7

24. Ice in the glass

Move 2 matchsticks and reform the glass in the same shape so the ice is outside it.

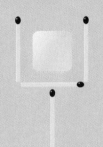

25. Doubling up

Move 1 match to make 4 triangles.

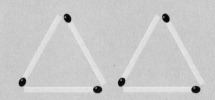

26. The elusive square

Move 1 match to make a square.

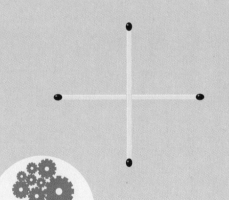

27. Two's company

Remove 2 matches to leave 2 squares.

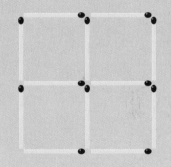

Sleeping on it

Did some of these matchstick puzzles baffle you? Perhaps what you should have done is slept on it. Have you ever had the experience of falling asleep after worrying for hours about some seemingly intractable problem, only to wake up the next morning with the perfect answer? Actually, the ability to sleep on a problem and solve it as if by magic is a common human trait.

How does it happen? It seems that as much as we need peaceful thinking time to create, our brain also appreciates the time to cogitate and deliver solutions while our consciousness is temporarily switched off. This may free the mind from the limitation imposed by ingrained beliefs. Sleep specialists don't know exactly at what point this unconscious search takes place, but it seems likely that it occurs during Rapid Eye Movement (REM) sleep, the period that is also associated with dreaming, and the retention of memories and learning (see p.42).

→ Original answers

A physics professor was about to give a university student a zero for an answer to a question on a test paper. The student argued that he should receive full credit, and blamed the system for refusing to recognize how well-informed his answer was. Finally, the teacher and student agreed to submit the paper to an impartial arbiter.

The examination problem was: "Show how it is possible to determine the height of a tall building using a barometer."

The student's answer was: "Take the barometer to the top of the building, attach a long rope to it, and lower the barometer to the ground. Then, bring it back up, measuring the length of the rope and the barometer. Add the two lengths and you will get the height of the building."

Second attempt

The arbiter pointed out that although the student had answered the problem correctly, his answer did not demonstrate any knowledge of physics so he couldn't be awarded any credit. He then suggested that the student make another attempt.

He was given six minutes to answer the same question, with the warning that this time the answer should indicate some knowledge of physics. At the end of five minutes, the student claimed he had several answers and was trying to select the best one. He then dashed off the following answer: "Take the barometer to the top of the building. Lean over the edge of the roof, drop the barometer, and time its descent with a stopwatch. Then, using the formula $S=\frac{1}{2}at^2$, calculate the height of the building. The arbiter decided to award him a good mark since he had demonstrated some knowledge of physics.

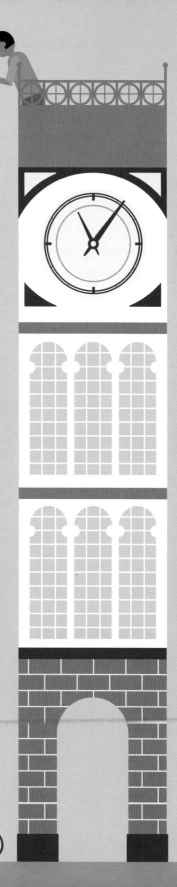

Alternative answers

Recalling the student had mentioned having alternative answers, the arbiter then asked him what they were. The student replied:

1. Take the barometer out on a sunny day and measure the height of the barometer, the length of its shadow, and the length of the building's shadow, then use simple proportion to determine the height of the building.

2. Take the barometer and begin to walk up the stairs. As you climb, mark off lengths of the barometer along the wall, then count the number of marks to get the height of the building in barometer units.

3. Tie the barometer to the end of a string, swing it and determine the value of the *"gyromagnetic-factor."* The building's height can be calculated from this value.

4. Take the barometer to the basement and knock on the owner's door. Then offer the barometer as a gift only if the owner tells you the building's height. (Although this solution doesn't show any knowledge of physics, it does make use of the barometer.)

Noticing that the arbiter wasn't too impressed with the last of those solutions, the student reluctantly admitted that he even knew the correct textbook answer:

5. Measure the air pressure at the bottom and top of the building and then apply the proper formula, illustrating that pressure decreases as height increases.

However, the student told the arbiter that he was so fed up with college professors trying to teach him how to think that he had decided to rebel.

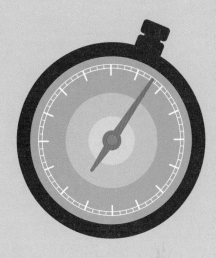

28. Polar explorer

Now that you know that there are many correct ways to answer a test question, try finding a solution to the question below:

Scott Amundsen Peary, the extravagantly named Polar explorer, claimed that when he was in the far North, he could point his car north on an ordinary road, drive it for 1 mile, and without turning around, end up 1 mile south of where he started. How did he do it?

solution on p.177 ⟫

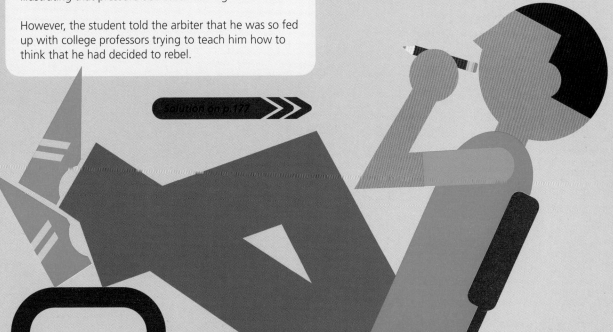

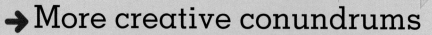

→ More creative conundrums

Although the following riddles do have a definitive answer, which can be found in the solutions section at the back of the book, it doesn't mean that other explanations are not possible, if not more plausible. Your imagination might actually take you in a totally different direction. If so, run with it! See where your creativity takes you. It might be that your explanation is a lot more interesting than the one we offer. What's more, you might think the answer we've given is, frankly, a bit silly.

29. A son's gratitude

A man locked his son out of the house.
The son thanked him. Explain.

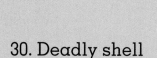

30. Deadly shell

The ancient Greek playwright Aeschylus was killed by a tortoise. How?

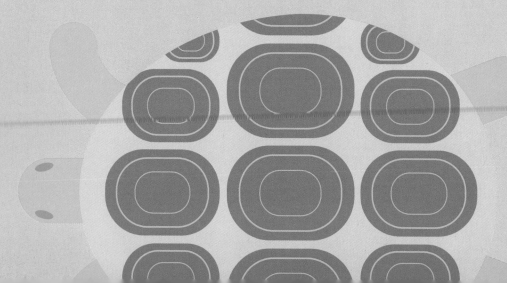

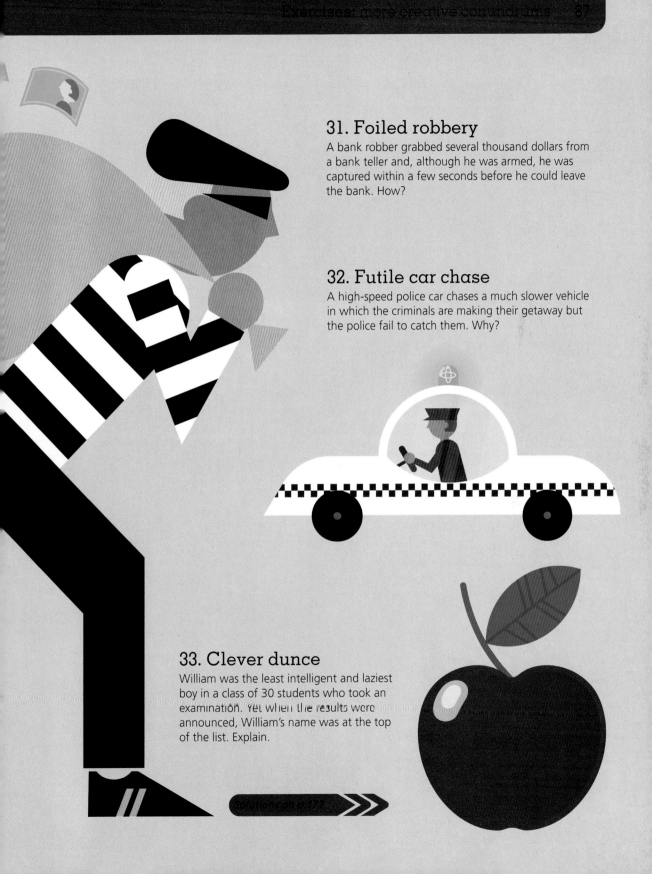

31. Foiled robbery

A bank robber grabbed several thousand dollars from a bank teller and, although he was armed, he was captured within a few seconds before he could leave the bank. How?

32. Futile car chase

A high-speed police car chases a much slower vehicle in which the criminals are making their getaway but the police fail to catch them. Why?

33. Clever dunce

William was the least intelligent and laziest boy in a class of 30 students who took an examination. Yet when the results were announced, William's name was at the top of the list. Explain.

Solutions on p.177

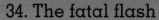

34. The fatal flash

There is a flash of light and a man dies. The man is not killed by any other person, a bolt of lightning, nor does he die of any illness, such as a heart attack. It's not suicide either. Can you suggest a plausible explanation?

35. Lax borders

An ordinary American citizen, with no passport, visits more than 30 foreign countries in one day. He is welcomed into each country and leaves each one of his own volition. How is that possible?

36. Strange detour

A man lives on the 10th floor of a building. Every day he takes the elevator to the first floor to go to work or to go shopping. When he returns he takes the elevator to the 7th floor and walks up the stairs to reach his apartment on the 10th floor. The man hates walking, so why does he do it?

37. Bottled money

If you put a small coin into an empty wine bottle and replace the cork, how would you get the coin out of the bottle without taking out the cork or breaking the bottle?

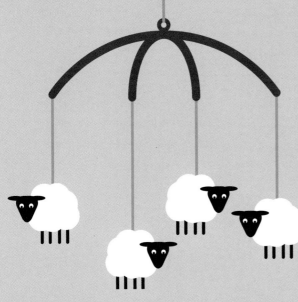

38. Separated at birth?

A woman had two sons who were born on the same hour of the same day of the same year. But they were not twins. How could this be so?

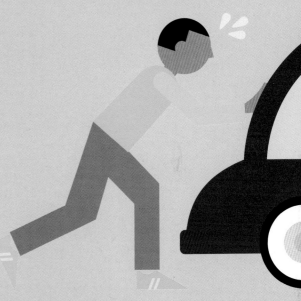

39. Push that car

A man pushed his car. He stopped when he reached a hotel, at which point he knew he was bankrupt. Why?

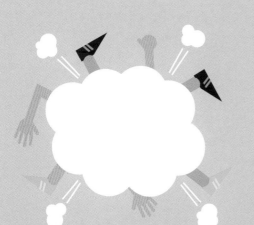

40. Newspaper divider

Tom and his younger sister were fighting. Their mother decided to punish them by making them stand on the same sheet of newspaper in such a way that they couldn't touch each other. How did she accomplish this?

41. Nail on the tree

When John was 6 years old he hammered a nail into his favorite tree to mark his height. Ten years later, at age 16, John returned to see how much higher the nail was. If the tree grew by 2 inches each year, how much higher would the nail be?

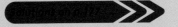

Solutions on p.177

→ Optical illusions

Optical illusions offer a great insight into how your creative mind works. They prove that the eye doesn't really see but merely collects information that it passes down to the brain, where innumerable processes of analysis, association, and qualification begin. Therein lies your creative powerhouse. Making sense of an image is one of the most creative acts the human brain engages in. Your brain essentially recreates the world on the canvas of your mind. In this creative process, the eyes are merely functionary. They simply deliver the raw material to your brain.

That's why the study of visual illusions and mental fallacies is useful. While they point out the limits of perception, they also reveal the magic your creative consciousness is capable of. Some illusions teach us to doubt and to question the many appearances of reality, while others, such as stereogram drawings (popularly known as Magic Eye), ask you to make sense of seemingly random elements.

Optical illusions can act as great creative stimulators because they are visual, engage the right-hand side of the brain, and force you to see things differently as you attempt to work out just what is happening.

42. The café wall
Are the horizontal lines on the wall parallel to each other or tapering?

43. Big-headed flower
By looking at the two flower heads, can you guess which central circle is larger: the one on the left or the one on the right?

44. Confused creature
What animal can you see, a duck or a rabbit?

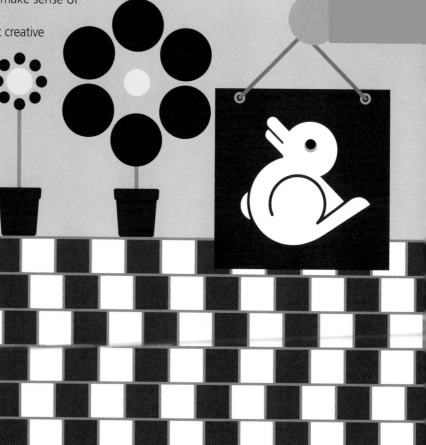

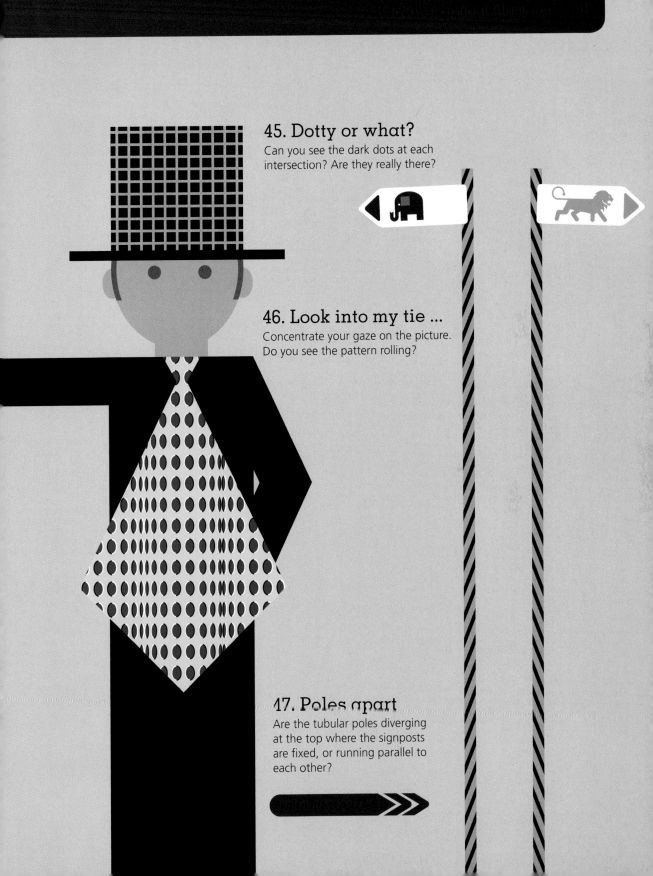

45. Dotty or what?
Can you see the dark dots at each intersection? Are they really there?

46. Look into my tie ...
Concentrate your gaze on the picture. Do you see the pattern rolling?

47. Poles apart
Are the tubular poles diverging at the top where the signposts are fixed, or running parallel to each other?

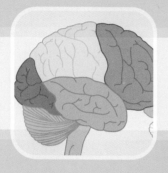

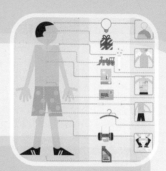

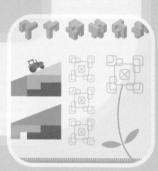

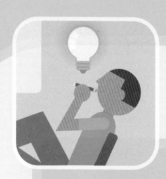

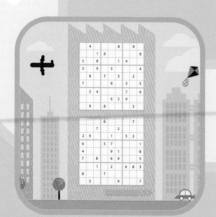

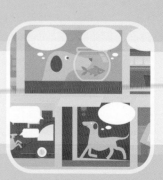

Chapter 5
Numerical reasoning

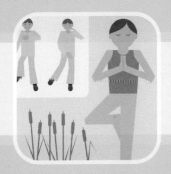

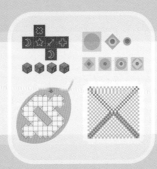

Numerical aptitude

Numbers are everywhere! But mention mathematics and many of us cower. That may be surprising since even babies and animals can register some kind of rudimentary counting mechanism. Everyone has an innate degree of numerical aptitude. It's built into our nature. We are always handling numbers and performing mental exercises with them. Think about it. When we wake up, it is usually because our alarm clock goes off at a set time—a time that we interpret through reading numbers. When we buy something, we quantify its value with the help of numbers. When we make our favorite dish following a recipe in a book, we use numbers to get the proportions of the ingredients right. Numerical reasoning forms the cornerstone of logic, rationality, argument, and proof. Yet, when many of us are asked whether we are any good at math, we tend to answer in the negative because the word dredges up memories of struggling with formulas and fractions, geometry and trigonometry. Why is this?

"Everyone has an innate degree of numerical aptitude. It's built into our nature. We are always handling numbers and performing mental exercises with them."

Numerophobia

Some people have difficulty dealing with numbers from a young age. Whether it's caused by a fear that developed at school or is some kind of mental block, they cannot cope. If you're one of them, you might be someone who suffers from numerophobia: literally, the fear of numbers—an irrational belief that your brain cannot process mathematical problems (although math is about applying logic and rationality, it is, paradoxically, affected by emotion). The truth is that even those of you who suffer from the phobia still apply mathematical skills unconsciously throughout your daily life. Overcoming the anxiety requires an ongoing commitment to learning, to acknowledging fears and working through them. You'll be surprised how quickly the brain learns new responses to enduring fears.

Visualizing math

Numerical reasoning becomes easier when you visualize mathematical concepts. Einstein once claimed that his thinking process took place through visualization and that he very rarely thought in words at all. Crucially, brain scans show that during calculations activity is not confined to the left hemisphere, but is also present in the visual, auditory, and motor areas of the brain. Furthermore, geometry and reading graphs by their nature require you to use your visual skills to understand complex numerical data, which immediately involves regions of the right temporal lobe. What we do know is that when a math problem is presented visually, it becomes clearer and more accessible, and the brain is more capable of recalling the knowledge later on.

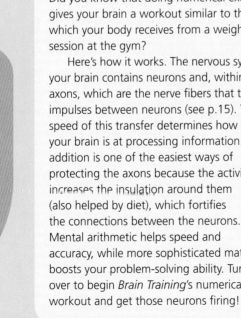

Number workout

Did you know that doing numerical exercises gives your brain a workout similar to that which your body receives from a weight session at the gym?

Here's how it works. The nervous system of your brain contains neurons and, within them, axons, which are the nerve fibers that transfer impulses between neurons (see p.15). The speed of this transfer determines how efficient your brain is at processing information. Doing addition is one of the easiest ways of protecting the axons because the activity increases the insulation around them (also helped by diet), which fortifies the connections between the neurons. Mental arithmetic helps speed and accuracy, while more sophisticated math boosts your problem-solving ability. Turn over to begin *Brain Training*'s numerical workout and get those neurons firing!

→ Quick-fire arithmetic test

Below are some problems to test your aptitude for basic arithmetic. The key is to do these in the quickest time possible without a calculator. Mental arithmetic is a robust mental exercise, accessing the powers of your short-term memory together with your ability to solve problems.

1. 3 + 9 + 7 =
a. 17
b. 18
c. 19

2. 13 – 5 =
a. 8
b. 7
c. 9

3. 25 – 16 =
a. 9
b. 11
c. 8

4. 9 x 7 =
a. 56
b. 63
c. 72

5. 9 x 8 x 2 =
a. 144
b. 156
c. 125

6. 66 ÷ 11 =
a. 6
b. 9
c. 8

7. 120 ÷ 4 ÷ 6 =
a. 7
b. 5
c. 12

8. 329 + 457 =
a. 786
b. 820
c. 790

9. 60 – (36 ÷ (3 x 4)) =
a. 98
b. 57
c. 32

10. Which of the following gives the answer 510?
a. 5 x 2 x 43
b. 2 x 5 x 51 x 7
c. 2 x 3 x 5 x 17

11. $^{50}/_{250}$ reduced to its lowest fraction term is:
a. $^{2}/_{13}$
b. $^{1}/_{5}$
c. $^{3}/_{7}$

12. 6.6 ÷ 2.2 =
a. 3
b. 3.3
c. 2.2

13. Which of the following gives the answer 560?
a. 20 x 30 – 30
b. 20 x 25 + 60
c. 20 x 29 – 25

14. 150 x 9 =
a. 1532
b. 1350
c. 1575

15. 15% of 35 =
a. 6
b. 6.5
c. 5.25

16. The answer to this calculation in its lowest terms is:
$^{20}/_{40} + ^{2}/_{8} =$
a. $^{3}/_{4}$
b. $^{1}/_{8}$
c. $^{12}/_{3}$

17. 4.6 + 0.23 + 1.96 =
a. 1.46
b. 2.63
c. 6.79

18. 195 ÷ 5 =
a. 38
b. 39
c. 40

19. 103 – 2.68 =
a. 100.42
b. 99.68
c. 100.32

20. 6¼ x 6 =
a. $^{2}/_{5}$
b. 37½
c. 37⅕

21. In lowest fraction terms express 40 minutes of three hours.
a. $^{6}/_{16}$
b. $^{5}/_{12}$
c. $^{2}/_{9}$

22. 6% of 230 =
a. 138
b. 13.8
c. 1.38

23. (-6) – (+3) =
a. 3
b. -3
c. -9

24. 250 X 7 =
a. 1750
b. 1850
c. 1950

25. 8% of 400 =
a. 50
b. 52
c. 32

26. 260 ÷ 5 =
a. 50
b. 52
c. 56

27. 15% of 70 =
a. 10.5
b. 11
c. 9

28. 168 x 9 =
a. 1512
b. 1550
c. 1580

29. 114 − 12.68 − 1.32 =
a. 100.42
b. 100
c. 100.32

30. Which of the following gives the answer 1536?
a. 8 x 6 x 32
b. 6 x 3 x 10
c. 9 x 5 x 35

31. 7.75 x 8 =
a. 60
b. 61
c. 62

32. 6% of 300 =
a. 16
b. 18
c. 20

33. 5 x 6 x 3 ÷ 5 =
a. 18
b. 22
c. 24

34. (-9) + (-22) =
a. -13
b. 13
c. -31

35. 60 x 3 + 20 ÷ 5 =
a. 50
b. 45
c. 40

How did you do?

This is math without any visual aid and you probably relied on the things you've learned by rote to answer the multiplication and division questions. Basic arithmetic benefits from frequent practice and repetition. Turn over and learn some killer tips to improve your numerical skills.

Men and women

So is it true that men perform better at mathematical subjects than women? Stereotypically, people tend to believe that the answer is "yes." However, most statistics show that female students perform on average at exactly the same level as their male counterparts all the way through school, so the real answer to the question is "no."

Until, that is to say, you get above and beyond higher education. At this point, it is true that most of the mathematical geniuses tend to be men: Archimedes, Newton, Einstein, Hawking. You get the picture.

Why is this? Perhaps more men choose to spend their adult lives refining their aptitude for numeracy. Perhaps women have not been encouraged enough in the past so it's down to historical conditioning. Perhaps now, with gender equality, we will see a few female mathematical geniuses join the ranks.

Time taken: *N°. correct answers:*

mins

/35

All correct under 3 mins excellent
3–4 mins—very good
over 4 mins—keep practicing

Solutions on p.178 >>

→ Improving numeracy

The key to improving your numerical skills is constant practice. The first thing to do if you're serious about improving your general mental arithmetic is to stop relying on your calculator. Of course, a calculator is a very useful and necessary tool. The trouble is that it allows such a large part of both sides of your brain to become just a little lazy. So if you want to improve arithmetic skills, you need to do without a calculator for all basic arithmetic calculations.

Another thing to remember is that improving your mathematical skills gives you a great mental pay off—it produces an instant buzz. When you get it, you feel clever. Math beyond basic arithmetic, such as geometry, incorporates powerful visualization skills because you have to use your mind's eye to arrive at the answer. Keep practicing and your ability to concentrate will become stronger. As a consequence, your overall capabilities in all other areas will improve; you will become more focused, which is a key factor in becoming successful in life.

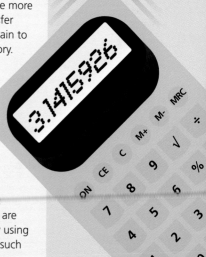

Tips

• Take your time, especially if you're out of practice. Think of it as a process to improve your aptitude rather than a test you need to pass in the quickest time. Speed will come with practice and understanding the mathematical process.

• Be imaginative with math. Try to see a problem in different ways. This will allow you to use a range of different methods to arrive at the answer. Opposite are a few shortcuts that will be helpful if you repeat the quick-fire test.

• To develop your ability to perform quick calculations, include numerical testers into your daily life. Add up grocery bills in your head as you go around the store. If you drive, calculate in your head how much you'll have to pay for a quarter, half, three-quarters, and full tank of fuel. Next time you're in a restaurant with friends, don't use the calculator on your mobile phone; instead, use mental arithmetic to figure out how much each of you will owe.

• Once you understand a concept, keep practicing. This is important since the more you practice, the more the concept will transfer from your working brain to your long-term memory.

• Visualize! It is a natural function of the mind and should be applied to many mathematical tasks. Key concepts such as division or place value (100s, 10s, and units) are often made clearer by using pictorial explanations such as graphs and tables.

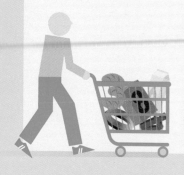

Shortcuts

Multiplying by 9: if you have to multiply a number in your head by 9, let's say 168: multiply it by 10 (1,680) and take away 168, giving the answer: 1,512.

Adding big numbers: if you have to add some fairly tricky numbers in your head, for example 329 and 457, round one of the numbers up (329 to 330), making a total of 787 easier to calculate, then subtract 1 to get the answer of 786.

15 percent tip: if you need to leave a 15% tip after a meal at a restaurant, here's an easy way to do it. Work out 10% (divide the number by 10)—then add that number to half its value and you have your answer.
15% of $35 = (10% of 35) + ((10% of 35) ÷ 2)
$3.50 + $1.75 = $5.25

Percentages: find 7% of 300. Sounds tricky? First of all, think about the words, "percent"—it means per hundred. So, it follows that 7 percent of 100 is 7; 8% of 100 = 8; 35.73% of 100 = 35.73. But how is that useful?

Back to the 7% of 300 question. 7% of the 1st hundred is 7. 7% of the 2nd hundred is also 7, and yes, 7% of the 3rd hundred is also 7. So 7 + 7 + 7 = 21. If 8% of 100 is 8, it follows that 8% of 50 is half of 8, or 4.

Dividing by 5: dividing a large number by 5 is actually very simple. All you do is multiply the number by 2 and move the decimal point: 2978 ÷ 5.
Step 1: 2978 x 2 = 5956
Step 2: 595.6

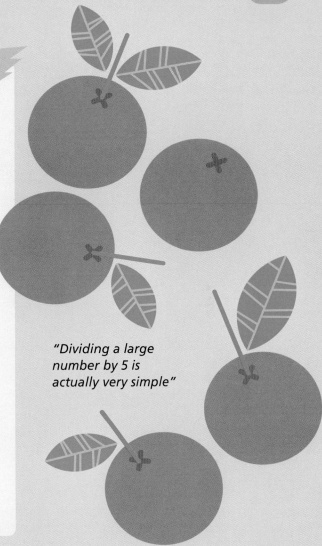

"Dividing a large number by 5 is actually very simple"

Pie charts

Pie charts are an easy way to visualize percentages. They are useful for analyzing polls and statistics, and managing time or money.

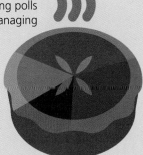

Life before the mobile memory

Can you recall the days when you had to keep a memory of all the phone numbers that were important to you? Today it's easy just to click on someone's name, press the green button, and let the handset do the rest. But what happens if you lose your handset and haven't kept a written record of the numbers? Yes, you're stuck! Why not take yourself back to those days when people had to store numbers in their heads? Try to memorize as many phone numbers as you can. OK, it's essentially a memory exercise, but you'll be amazed how the constant calling to mind of different numbers improves your numerical skills, especially your aptitude for mental arithmetic.

Visual math workout

Different parts of your brain become active once you start making math visual, which leads to a more holistic brain workout. In addition, you learn to understand the language of mathematics by finding ways to visualize its logical meaning. The truth is, many people are instantly put off by a numerical problem when it is presented with large numbers and arcane symbols. So it stands to reason that adding a visual component to learning math makes it more engaging from the start.

   Below is an example to get you started. If you simply read the problem, you might become confused because of the information "overload" but the problem becomes much easier when you study the diagram below. Afterward, try the other visual exercises on the next few pages.

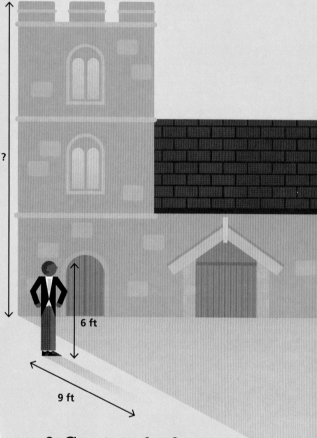

1. Under the bridge

An aerial photograph was taken of a bus passing under a bridge. In the picture, part of the bus has traveled past the bridge. One half of the bus is yet to cross under the bridge. Two-thirds of the other half of the bus is directly under the bridge; and 9 ft of it has passed the bridge.

How long is the bus?

____ ft

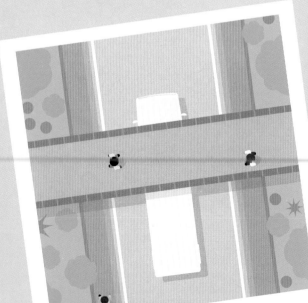

2. Casting shadows

It is a sunny day. Steve, who is 6 ft tall, casts a shadow that is 9 ft long (see above).

A: How tall is the building behind him if it casts a shadow that is 135 ft?

____ ft

B: Three hours later, Steve's shadow increases to 13½ ft. What is the length of the shadow the building is casting now?

____ ft

Solutions on p.178 ⟫⟫

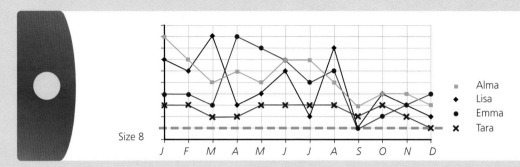

Size 8

J F M A M J J A S O N D

■ Alma
◆ Lisa
● Emma
✕ Tara

3. Wedding fit

Alma, Lisa, Emma, and Tara are friends whose boyfriends proposed to them on the same day. They are all getting married in 18 months' time, and they would all like to fit into a size-8 dress. They each diet and begin an exercise program. Their first years' progress toward their ideal weight is shown above.

A: In which month did Alma and Emma's size differ the most?

B: Whose weight was most consistent throughout the year?

C: Which bride will fit into a size-8 dress after 12 months?

4. Chance amour

In an art gallery, two strangers take a fancy to each other. They are 120 ft apart. The man walks toward the woman at a rate of 9 ft/sec. The woman plays it cool, edging toward the man at 3 ft/sec.

How long before they meet?

secs

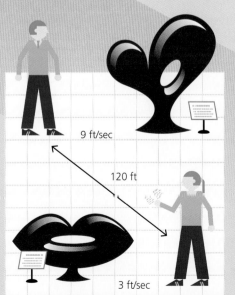

9 ft/sec

120 ft

3 ft/sec

5. Keen student

Jack walks to the bus stop to catch a bus to his university. He then walks from the bus stop at the university to the student center, arriving there at 9:35 am.

A: How far does Jack walk in total?

miles

B: How far is he from the university student center at 9:20am?

miles

C: What is the average speed of the bus?

mph

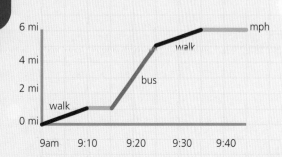

6 mi

4 mi

2 mi

0 mi

mph

walk

bus

walk

mph

9am   9:10   9:20   9:30   9:40

6. Carrying cupcakes

Philippa is holding a tea party in her garden and is offering her hungry guests cupcakes on different size trays. The cupcakes she has made measure 2 x 2 in.

How many cupcakes can she fit side by side on each of the trays illustrated in the picture?

Small tray: *cakes*

Medium tray: *cakes*

Large tray: *cakes*

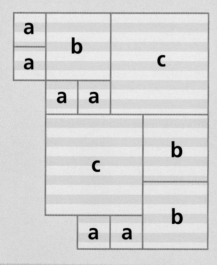

12 in
8 in

16 in
10 in

16 in
12 in

7. Land up for grabs

Farmer Giles has decided to sell off his allotment. He divides the land into 3 different size plots: "a," "b," and "c." The dimensions of his plots are shown below.

a   12 x 12 ft

b   24 x 24 ft

c   36 x 36 ft

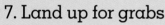

A: What is the total amount of land in feet that Farmer Giles owns?   *ft²*

B: An interested client only wants to buy the "c" plots. What is the total area of that land?   *ft²*

C: Another client opts to buy all the "a" and "c" plots. How much land is that in total?   *ft²*

D: The plots cost $2,000 per 900 ft². How much are all the "b" plots worth? $

E: A client offers to buy all the plots. What is the total price he'll be asked to pay? $

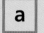
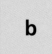

Solutions on p.178

8. Bathroom makeover

A: Philip is tiling his bathroom wall. The diagram shows how much he has completed. Write down as a fraction in its lowest terms how much he has left to tile.

B: The tiles come in packs of 8. How many packs will he need to tile the white wall?

packs

C: Each pack costs $2.40. How much will it cost him to tile the wall?

$

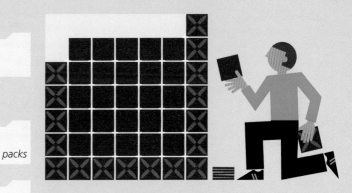

9. Computer sales

This graph gives the number of computers sold each month (in hundreds) by 3 different computer manufacturers:
Manufacturer 1 (in red)
Manufacturer 2 (in blue)
Manufacturer 3 (in green).

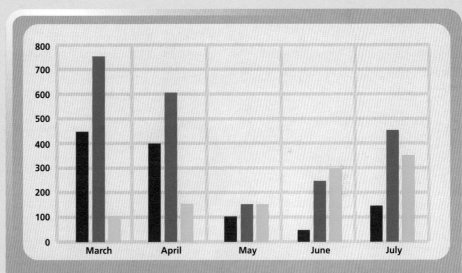
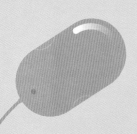

A: Which month showed the largest total decrease in PC sales since the previous month?

B: What percentage of Manufacturer 2's sales was made in April (to the nearest percent?

C: How many units did Manufacturer 3 sell over the five months?

%

Does faster equal smarter?

If you're able to think more quickly does that make you a smarter person than someone who takes more time? In general terms, we'd have to say it's debatable. For example, an artist may take years working on a masterpiece but does that reflect on his or her intelligence? In numerical terms, however, the answer is "yes." The speed in which you managed to complete these exercises is an indication of your current numerical aptitude. The ability to process information rapidly indicates there is more neuron activity in those areas of the brain. However, you should always take enough time to ensure that the answers are correct. It's not very smart to make mistakes through sheer carelessness.

finish

10. The shortest route

The objective is to create a path that starts in the lower left corner and ends in the upper right corner. Each number represents the distance in feet of the line it is on.

Your goal is to find the shortest path possible through the grid. We've given you a head start. Can you finish it?

Your score:

Time taken:

mins

```
   8 — 3 — 6 — 7 — 8 — 7 — 5 — 2
 7   8   7   6   5   5   8   7   1
   2 — 7 — 2 — 4 — 6 — 6 — 5 — 2
 1   3   2   1   9   9   3   1   3
   8 — 4 — 9 — 4 — 6 — 7 — 6 — 5
 4   6   5   4   3   3   5   2   4
   4 — 2 — 8 — 4 — 7 — 9 — 1 — 9
 5   7   7   6   4   4   6   3   4
   9 — 8 — 7 — 3 — 8 — 2 — 4 — 5
 5   8   8   7   5   5   6   3   3
   2 — 3 — 3 — 1 — 7 — 3 — 6 — 8
 4   7   7   6   5   4   5   1   1
   9 — 2 — 4 — 4 — 3 — 9 — 5 — 9
 2   5   6   5   3   2   3   8   7
   1 — 5 — 9 ┌ 2 — 2 — 1 — 8 — 5
 7   2   3   2   9   8   9   4   3
   3 — 1 — 7 ┘ 2 — 4 — 5 — 5 — 4
```

start

11. The broken calculator

This calculator fell out of your bag and into a puddle, and is now experiencing a major malfunction. Only the buttons highlighted in the picture actually work.
Your task is to compute the numbers 1 through to 15 with the limited means the calculator offers. For instance, 0.5 x 2 will give you "1"—the first of the 15 digits.

Can you use your mental arithmetic skills to figure out the remaining numbers?

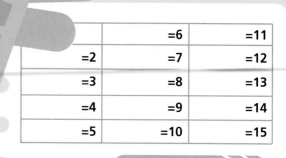

		=6		=11
	=2		=7	=12
	=3		=8	=13
	=4		=9	=14
	=5		=10	=15

Solutions on p.179 »»

12. Unfold the folds

A piece of paper has been folded 5 times with a single straight fold down the middle so that the edges line up. Folded, its dimensions measure 7 x 4 in.

Calculate its original dimensions

in

Hint: visualize the unfolding pattern.

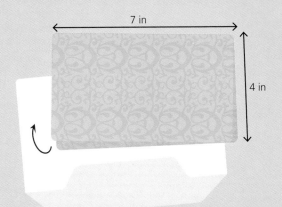

7 in

4 in

13. Triangle ratio

A circle has an equilateral triangle touching its circumference on the outside and another equilateral triangle touching its circumference on the inside, as pictured.

What is the ratio of the areas of these two triangles?

:

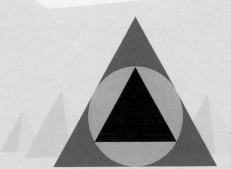

14. Cross math

Fill the empty cells with the correct number or function.

					2				2	
				8	÷		=	4	+	
	3		7		1					
		+			=		4	x		= 4
	9	x	8	=			x		8	
	=						0			
	1		1	+		− 6	=			9
5	2		2		+		0	5		÷
x			=		3			÷		3
	−		= 3		=		4	5	÷	= 5
−								=		x
4	÷					+	3	= 6		7
0	7									=
	=									
						1 2	−		=	

Career with no math?

So you might be wondering how these math exercises could relate to your everyday life. The familiar story is that we leave school or college and consign our math books to the attic, or even throw them away, thankful that we won't have to do another calculation for the rest of our days. Think again! Do you know how many jobs or careers exist where you won't have to use what math you have learned? On average, less than 10 percent throughout the world (and even that estimate is a very conservative one)

The truth is that everybody needs to use numerical skills at every stage, whether in personal or working lives, and the more well-honed yours are, the better.

Sudoku

Over the last few years, Sudoku has become one of the most popular games worldwide for exercising your brain. Although popularized in Japan during the mid-1980s, it was actually invented by an American, Howard Garns, in 1979, and was then called Number Place.

It is a neat little puzzle consisting of nine squares with nine spaces in each square, which are so placed as to form one large square, with vertical and horizontal lines, each with nine spaces. The aim is to fill in a 9 x 9 grid of 81 cells, subdivided into 3 x 3 subgrids, with the numbers 1–9. Each digit can appear only once in each column, row, and subgrid. The whole puzzle is based on what is known as a Latin square, possibly a reference to the preferred Roman military formation.

Sudoku is a logic exercise. It uses numbers but the puzzle involves no arithmetic as such. Following the rules of the game, and using the numbers already given, you work out what the other numbers must be through a process of deduction. The great thing about Sudoku is that each successful step makes the next step easier by narrowing the possibilities. Every box you solve offers a clue to fill another box.

Rules of Sudoku at a glance:

• Each box (subgrid) of nine squares must contain the numbers 1 to 9, each appearing once only.
• So must each column of nine square.
• So must each row of nine squares.

2	5	7	4	8	1	9	6	3
1	9	3	6	2	7	5	4	8
8	4	6	5	3	9	1	7	2
3	6	1	7	5	8	2	9	4
9	8	5	1	4	2	7	3	6
7	2	4	9	6	3	8	5	1
6	3	2	8	7	5	4	1	9
4	7	9	2	1	6	3	8	5
5	1	8	3	9	4	6	2	7

column

row

subgrid

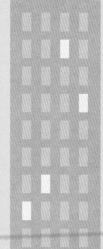
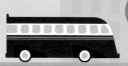
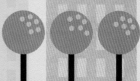

Easy Sudoku

The grids below are for the Sudoku virgins. As with all numerical reasoning games, you'll be amazed how much a little practice will improve your problem-solving skills.

All you experts will probably find these starter exercises a little easy. However, that doesn't mean you should ignore them altogether. You might want to boost your confidence by doing these puzzles first and finishing them in a ridiculously short time.

The grids become progressively more difficult on the next page. Don't worry though, we've given a few hints to help you with these. They also become much easier with practice.

You'll soon understand why Sudoku is so popular, especially if you are the kind of person who always likes to solve puzzles you begin—there's definitely some comfort in knowing that there is always a right answer. So, what are you waiting for? Get started!

Grid A

Grid B

Solutions on p.179

Intermediate Sudoku

Hint: one of the best pieces of advice is to "eliminate": look for spaces where numbers can't go. For instance, if a box has 4 unfilled spaces, but you see 3 of the remaining numbers won't go into one of those spaces, then the 4th number must go there.

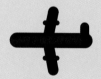

Grid C

	4				8		9	
		1	6					8
5		8			1	4		
3		9		5				4
	8		7		3		2	
7				8		3		5
	3	4				7		6
			6	2	9			
	9		8				3	

Grid D

			6				7	
		7			2			
2	9			1		5	3	
6			5	7				1
4				9	1			8
7		8		6	4			5
		1		2		6	8	3
8			7					
	3				9			7

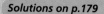

Solutions on p.179

Hard Sudoku

Hint: group possible numbers into pairs. If 2 will slot into a couple of spaces but you're not sure which goes where, pencil them in anyway. This might leave you a space where another number must fit through trial and error. These puzzles demand patience and perseverance.

Grid E

	8			3			4	
					2		3	
6			4	7				1
	5		2			8		
	3						9	
		2		3		5		
1			3	4				6
	7		9					
	4		2			7		

Age-proof the brain

The key to age-proofing the brain is to keep your brain active and to build on this. Simple techniques, such as games like Sudoku and the range of exercises in this book, challenge your brain and help keep it active. Think broad—if your work requires you to do the same kind of thing every day, try to learn a new skill, so your brain doesn't get lazy or inactive. (See Chapter 7 for more tips.)

Samurai Sudoku

The Samurai Sudoku is the monster puzzle that any Sudoku addict will, sooner or later, feel compelled to tackle. If you've enjoyed the Sudoku exercises, these should offer an excellent progression. The game is essentially the same as normal Sudoku except that it consists of five interlocking Sudoku grids, and will really call upon all your powers of concentration and deductive reasoning. And, of course, you'll get five times the satisfaction when you've solved the puzzle. Rumor has it that geishas invented these exercises to while away the long hours waiting for their Samurai lords to return from the battlefield—hence the name.

Grid A

Tips

• All normal rules for Sudoku apply: no number can be repeated in any row, column, or grid.

• The central grid is critical, since numbers in each of its four corners correspond to numbers in the corners of all the others.

• It's best to work inward from the outside grids; don't try to solve the central grid first.

• Concentrate on each grid briefly; keep moving clockwise before tackling the central grid.

• Don't allow yourself to be overwhelmed by the sheer scale of the puzzle; keep repeating your clockwise deductions.

Grid B

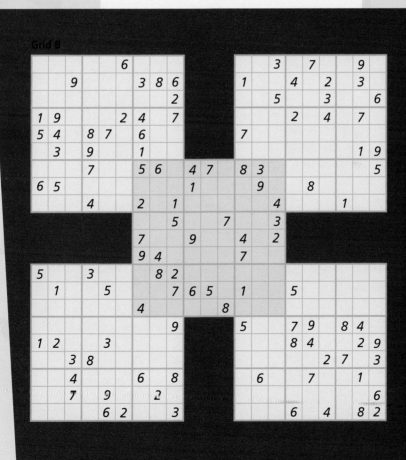

Solutions on p.180 >>>

→ Kakuro

Kakuro is the second most popular logic-puzzle game after Sudoku in Japan, and is also rapidly gaining the attention of puzzle fans throughout the world.

Kakuro is laid out slightly more like a crossword. Numbers, often called clues, are given in shaded squares, relating to the horizontal or vertical lines of numbers. Although a number can be used only once to make up each total sum, there is no such restriction over the puzzle as a whole, and consequently Kakuro solutions are less uniform and provide greater variety than those of Sudoku. Kakuro is a useful variant to Sudoku, since it not only tests your logical aptitude but also exercises your numerical reasoning skills because it demands that you use mental arithmetic to solve the puzzle.

It is this variety that tends to appeal to those who find Sudoku a little one-dimensional. Although starting off with obvious total combinations (4 = 1 + 3, 17 = 9 + 8), the answers have a greater impact upon each other, involving more combinations, and giving the final grid a very different feel. Since no numbers are filled in originally (unlike Sudoku), you often have to work out different combinations on a separate sheet, making it closer to the mathematics we all studied (or are studying) at school.

Rules of Kakuro at a glance:

• Each grid has a starting position like that of a crossword, containing shaded squares and blank squares, where you need to fill in a number from 1–9.
• In each blank square enter a number that adds up to the total stated for that column or row on the grid.
• No number may be repeated in making up any total.

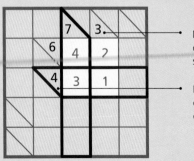

Numbers in the left lower part of each square refer to the total sum of the vertical column

Numbers in the right upper corner refer to the total sum of the horizontal row

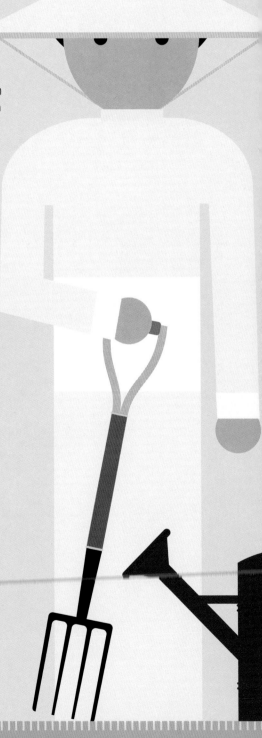

Kakuro games

Grid A: *Easy*

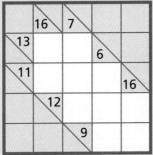

Grid B: *Easy*

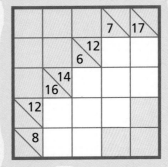

Grid C: *Moderate*

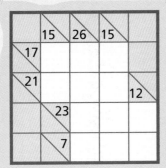

Grid D: *Moderate*

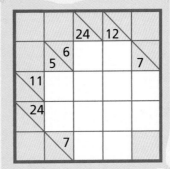

Grid E: *Hard*

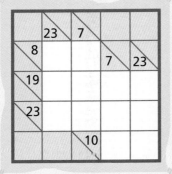

Grid F: *Hard*

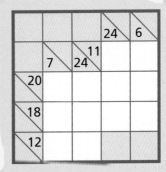

Solutions on p.180

Logic flies out of the window

OK, so you're now feeling more confident about using numbers and applying logic, both as a stimulus to mental activity and as a yardstick in everyday situations. But isn't there some nagging feeling in your psychological makeup that says: "Sure, these games may be useful at certain times but when it comes to things I know well, I've got my own trusted methods, thank you very much"? If you feel like this, then you're not alone.

Heuristics

At times, most of us resort to intelligent guesswork rather than logic which, in the field of psychology, is known as applying heuristic knowledge. This is a perfectly natural response to incomplete information or a complex problem. Our brains have been encoded with these generally efficient rules, either learned or inherited, which enable us to fill in the gaps. This is what leads us to make educated guesses and intuitive judgments. In other words, we are applying common sense. There's only one slight flaw—although our brains may lead us to the correct answer most of the time, they might also lead us astray unless we stop, take a step back, and apply logic. However, in practice this is easier said than done!

   The trouble is that although we are in the wrong and biased, we still believe that we're in the right. It's a recipe for trouble, which is why psychologists are so interested in the uses and effects of heuristics. Have a look at these examples. What would you think or do?

15. Lottery numbers

You go into the store to play the lottery because it's a rollover month and the jackpot is mammoth. The lady in front of you is also playing the lottery and she's marked down numbers: 1, 2, 3, 4, 5, 6. You think she's totally nuts for choosing those numbers because they'll never come up. Is she being ridiculous, or are you being illogical for entertaining that thought?

16. Beer money

You're on your way to meet friends and you find a $50 bill lying in the street. You pick it up and decide to buy everyone a drink with the money. In other words you're going to spend it on a whim. You attach less value to it than you would a $50 bill that you earned. Why so? Is it really worth any less?

Solutions on pp.180–1

17. Bidding war

You're at an antiques auction looking for new stock for your antiques shop. You've been flicking through the catalog and have spotted a beautiful carriage clock. When the lot comes up you start bidding, setting yourself a price limit. As the bidders fall away, there's one person left who keeps outbidding you. You glance over your shoulder to see that it is your arch competitor. Suddenly the price limit you set yourself means very little. Why are you being so illogical? Don't you have a business to run?

18. Expensive tastes

An inexpensive bottle of cologne costs $30, whereas a designer brand costs $60. The retailers increase the price of the cheaper scent to $65. Which do you think will sell more?

Conclusion

Turn to the back of the book for the explanations. You'll see that the logic is simple, but in certain situations these common biases can easily creep into our minds.

What conclusion can we draw from this? Well, occasionally it's fair to say that the human brain seems to want to let logic fly out of the window. It might even be the natural order of things. After all, it's only logical that we behave like human beings.

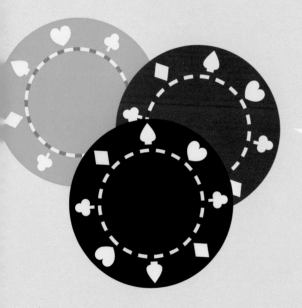

19. Bad luck?

You are with your friend in Las Vegas at a roulette table. Your friend has just won for the sixth time in succession by putting her chips on the red. She's becoming really smug while you're running out of chips. You challenge her to try again. She obliges and advises you to always put the chips on the red. You spite her and put your remaining chip on the black. Who do you think has a better chance of winning?

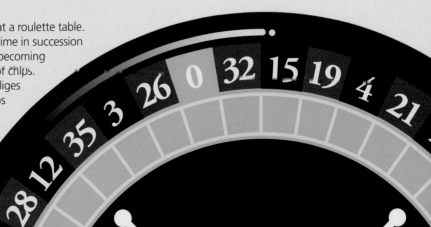

Gambler's fallacy

Bet you haven't heard examples of the gambler's mantra! Well, it goes like this: "the next horse is going to come first," or "the next card is going to be an ace," or "the next fruit is going to be that elusive third cherry." We all know that it doesn't really make sense, but the gambler conspires to kid himself that the fact he lost last time means that he's more likely to win next time. In reality, the dice are eternally loaded against us. Our chances are the same as before—pretty low, unfortunately. But don't tell that to the gambler. And certainly don't tell the person in front of you in the line who is about to play the lottery, because the odds for them are even worse. In fact, the odds of matching all six of six numbers from 49 are 1 in 18,069,460!

So, what makes us fly in the face of common sense? Why do gamblers play against the odds when they're often intelligent people? Is it just greed? Without going too deeply into psychological matters (basically, the driving force is being on the cusp of the unknown), the answer is that the lure of winning big overrides the gradual despondency of losing small—or even relatively large—over a period of time.

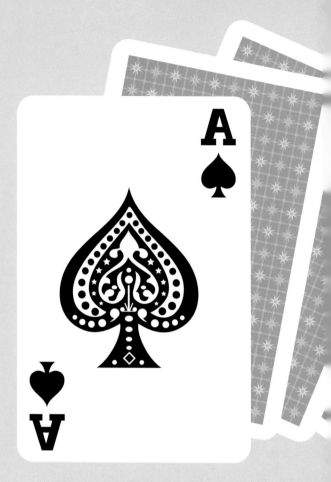

Looks good, sounds good, feels good!

The casinos and other gambling outlets are only too aware of this fallacy and do everything in their power to lure the gambler to part with that last coin rolling in his pocket. They resort to the theory of "affect heuristic" to influence the gambler's decision. What we mean by "affect" is that they offer multiple stimuli to generate an involuntary response. Slot machines are a perfect example. Think about all those flashing lights, the tantalizing colors, the pace at which the reels turn, the electronic sounds that imply you're on the brink of winning big. Oh, and what about that near miss? It's drawing you in, messing with your logic, and lowering your risk perception. It's manipulating you through your visual and aural senses. No wonder Las Vegas is the city of neon lights.

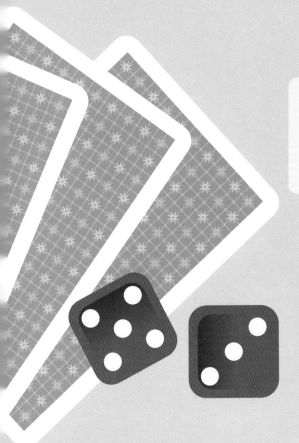

Sly, subtle scents

Did you know that many casino operators pump a scent into the air? This may sound rather bizarre, but in an experimental test the scent was shown to increase substantially the number of coins customers dropped into the slots—by about 45 percent!

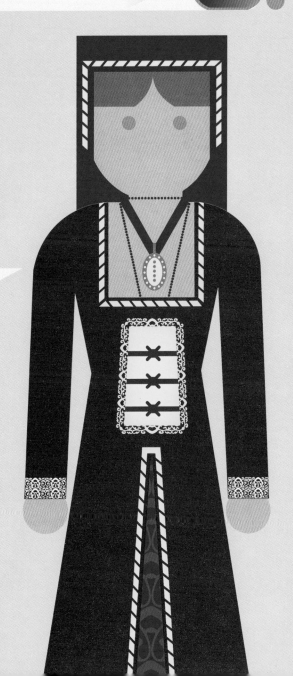

Law of averages

The law of averages is the diametric opposite of Murphy's Law. Basically, Murphy's Law states that if something can go wrong, it will, whereas the law of averages is usually invoked to say that if things haven't been going right, they will now. "By the law of averages, Katherine Howard is definitely the wife for me," said Henry VIII, the 16th-century king of England, delighting over his fifth marriage. Result: her execution a few months later. The law does not take into consideration other circumstances that might affect the outcome, and usually reflects bad statistics or wishful thinking rather than any mathematical principle.

20 Heads or tails?

Take a coin, and toss it, then flip it again, and so on. Write down how many times it comes down "heads" in the first 10 tosses. What are the odds of it being "heads" next time? Don't you dare fall for the heuristic impulse—you should know better by now!

Solution on p.181

Unraveling numerical riddles

Riddles are similar to logical fallacies (see pp.114–117) in that they make you employ false logic. Riddles are problems that are usually expressed in metaphorical or allegorical language, and are loaded with ambiguity. They are designed to trip you up, so you have to think carefully in order to find the correct solution.

The best riddles cause your brains to fill in the missing gaps without using sound reasoning, and they use all sorts of methods to lead you astray. Remember, mathematical riddles are abstract, so it's crucial to pay particular attention to information that doesn't seem important in the first reading. Some of the more "vital" information you are given might be there to lead you away from looking at the true problem itself!

Progression

Another common type of riddle involves numerical progression or a sequence of numbers. The tendency in the progression seems to be drawing you toward one answer, but in fact the answer lies elsewhere. Here's an example: 1, 1, 2, 3, 5...

Now, your initial instinct might be to propose this solution and the rest of the series of numbers based on prime numbers: 1, 1, 2, 3, 5, 7, 11, 13.

However, the correct answer is based on adding together the last two numbers (known as the Fibonacci sequence, after its inventor): 1, 1, 2, 3, 5, 8, 13, 21.

In this instance, the riddle has deceived you as to the type of progression used.

Misdirection

This is the standard ploy used in most riddles. Here's an example: "I have three coins in my pocket, which total 60 cents. Two of the coins are not quarters. What are the coins?"

The questioner invites you into all the byways of lateral thinking, but the answer depends on a trick. So before you start working out whether the question is referring to another currency or other complicated explanations, look at it again carefully.

"Two of the coins are not quarters." Sure, but the third one is. The answer is two quarters and a dime.

Logical teasers

We also include some logical conundrums, which offer apparently quirky answers to seemingly innocuous questions, brain teasers, and other mind twisters. This offshoot of math relies on thought rather than numbers. It tests your ability to figure out certain givens and connect them together until you arrive at the solution.

Question:

How do you get (exactly) 4 gallons of water out of a well if the only pieces of equipment you have are a 3-gallon bucket and a 5-gallon bucket?

Answer:

1. Fill the 5-gallon bucket from the well.
2. Use the 5-gallon bucket to fill up the 3-gallon bucket. This leaves 2 gallons in the 5-gallon bucket.
3. Empty the 3-gallon bucket into the well.
4. Pour the 2 gallons from the 5-gallon bucket into the 3-gallon bucket.
5. Fill up the 5-gallon bucket from the well.
6. Fill up the 3-gallon bucket using the 5-gallon bucket. The 3-gallon bucket already contains 2 gallons, so 1 gallon goes from the 5-gallon bucket to the 3-gallon bucket.
7. You have just removed 1 gallon from the 5-gallon bucket. Voila! That leaves you with 4 gallons.

→ Riddles to try

So, just for a bit of fun, take a look at these classic types of riddles. Don't worry too much if you need to peek at the answers—some of these are pretty difficult to solve. Of course, the more you practice, the easier they will become.

21. Number sequences

A: Find the next number in the following sequence:
1, 11, 21, 1211, 111221, 312211, ...

B: What's the next number in the sequence?
31, 28, 31, 30, 31, ...

C: Find the next number in the sequence:
1, 4, 1, 5, 9, 2, 6, ...

D: Find the next number in the sequence:
6, 25, 64, 81, 32 ...

Hint: just because you're presented with numbers doesn't mean that mathematical logic applies!

22. Chasing cars

Consider a road with 2 cars traveling toward each other with a distance of 100 miles between them. The left car travels at a speed of 40 mph and the right car at a speed of 60 mph. A bird starts at the same location as the right car and flies at a speed of 80 mph. When it reaches the left car it reverses direction, and when it reaches the right car it reverses again to the opposite, and so on.

What is the total distance that the bird has traveled at the moment the 2 cars have reached each other?

_____ miles

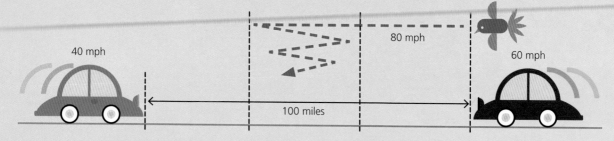

40 mph   80 mph   60 mph

100 miles

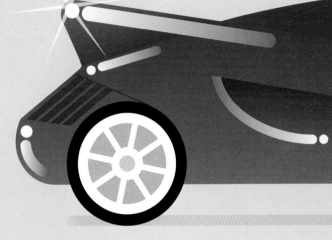

23. The famous 3 doors conundrum

You're appearing on a TV game show. The host shows you 3 closed doors and tells you that there is a flashy new red sportscar in a room behind one of them. The other rooms are empty. If you choose the correct door, you win it. You pick a door at random. The host, who knows where the car is, stops you, then opens another door and shows you an empty room. He asks if you want to change your mind. Should you?

yes   *no*

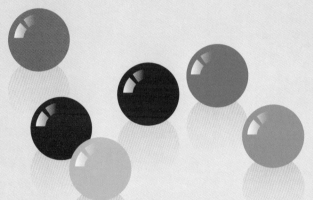

24. Weighing marbles

You have 10 bags with 10 marbles in each bag. All of the marbles weigh 1 oz except for the marbles in one bag, which weigh 0.9 oz. But you don't know which bag these 0.9 oz marbles are in. You have to find out by taking zero or more marbles from zero or more bags and putting them on weighing scales. After seeing the result of the weight, you should be able to tell which bag contains the marbles that weigh only 0.9 oz.

How many marbles from which bags do you take to weigh? (You'll need to work this out on a separate piece of paper.)

25. The condemned prisoner conundrum

You are one of 3 prisoners in the same cell condemned to death. The jailer capriciously decides that one of you may be spared—the one who's the first to guess correctly the color of the disk affixed to the back of his or her head. Any wrong guesses will mean instant death. The jailer shows all 3 of you that he has 5 disks: 2 black, 3 white. He uses 3 of them and hides the other 2. You can see that each of the other prisoners has a white disk.

What is the color of yours?

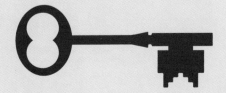

26. Break up time

Break this clock into (exactly) 5 pieces so that the sum of the numbers on each piece add up to 8, 10, 12, 14, and 16.

Hint: you're allowed to cut through double digits!

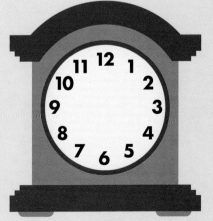

Solutions on pp.181–2

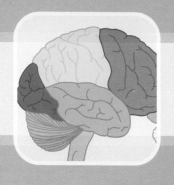

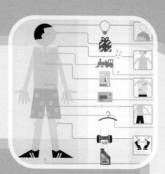

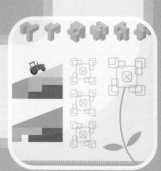

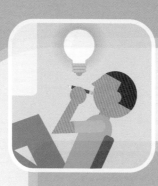

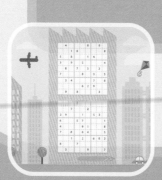

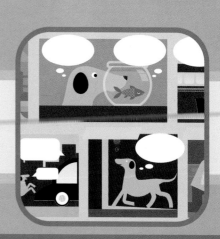

Chapter 6
Verbal reasoning

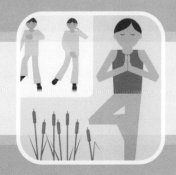
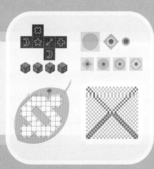

→ Talk your way to success

There is a direct correlation between verbal aptitude and success in life. We're not just talking about the ability to complete crosswords, unravel anagrams, or figure out antonyms, although all of those activities are great for exercising your verbal aptitude. We're talking more generally about the ability to use words, to manipulate language so that you can communicate ideas, thoughts, opinions, and feelings cogently. Arguably, politicians and lawyers utilize this skill best, as do rap artists and talk show hosts, who are all adept at engaging a mass audience with the power of words, often using them to influence an audience's way of thinking. In short, the better your verbal intelligence, the more confident you will be at asserting your needs and wants. You will be better understood and will be able to form closer relationships. Whatever the path you take in life, improving your verbal aptitude will have a marked effect on your social progress and prosperity.

Language and the visual

Scientists believe that by the age of five you may already have about 2,000 to 3,000 words in your vocabulary, but that does not mean you know the exact meaning of these words. For example, a child seeing a ball might say "ball" but he might also say "ball" pointing at a balloon, a chocolate egg, or a pebble. What this suggests is that on an instinctive level, the visual sense has an enormous influence on how language develops. For instance, consider the first alphabet book a child looks at. An image is used to qualify and give meaning to a character in an alphabet. For example, "A" for Apple, "B" for Bear, and so on, so it stands to reason that a young child uses the same word for similar-looking shapes until his vocabulary grows. And while you may think that this reliance upon the "visual" is something you grow out of by the time you get through school (having accumulated a

How it works

The ability to use words and tap into the vast possibilities of the spoken and written language boosts the brain's processing power by opening up additional neuron pathways. Scans have traced activity throughout the brain and not just the left side, indicating that verbal reasoning is an extremely complex process. When you engage in a conversation, a whole series of cognitive functions take place even before a sentence reaches the tip of your tongue. A thought lights up in your head, your brain then refines it using all the sensory associations, sends this information to two key areas of the brain (see below), which then select the necessary words to convey its meaning, and finally place the words into a grammatical framework. Only then are you ready to speak.

The language powerhouses

The two main powerhouses of the brain's linguistic system are called Wernicke's area and Broca's area, named after the two scientists who discovered these regions in the 1800s. Broca's area, which is located in the frontal lobe of the cortex, is responsible for language production—putting together sentences, using

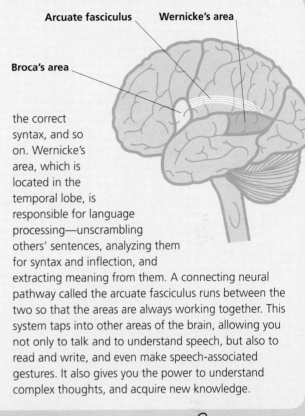

Arcuate fasciculus   **Wernicke's area**

Broca's area

the correct syntax, and so on. Wernicke's area, which is located in the temporal lobe, is responsible for language processing—unscrambling others' sentences, analyzing them for syntax and inflection, and extracting meaning from them. A connecting neural pathway called the arcuate fasciculus runs between the two so that the areas are always working together. This system taps into other areas of the brain, allowing you not only to talk and to understand speech, but also to read and write, and even make speech-associated gestures. It also gives you the power to understand complex thoughts, and acquire new knowledge.

vocabulary of about 50,000 words), consider the use of analogies, metaphors, and similes (see p.70). Visual concepts influence language throughout your life. For instance, public speakers and those in positions of power know that they stand a greater chance of keeping you engaged if they use words to tell a story that conjures up a "big picture." Words might evaporate, but use them to convey an image and the idea behind it will be more memorable. The great orators have always relied on the "visual" to fashion speeches. Consider Martin Luther King's famous address to the nation. The words "I have a dream..." instantly open a window to his vision of the future!

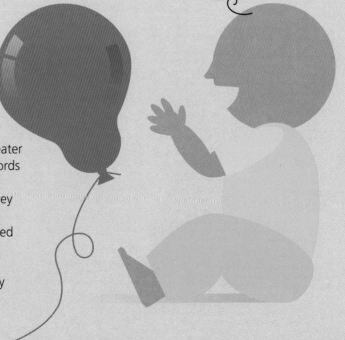

Quick-fire vocabulary test

We've grouped together a number of simple exercises to measure your current vocabulary. This is an example of the type of test a prospective employer might use to gauge an applicant's intelligence (and which forms part of psychometric testing). Admittedly, vocabulary exercises are a crude method and only test a specific branch of crystallized intelligence (see p.128), but since clear understanding and expression are necessary to most careers, any job selection process will inevitably test your vocabulary.

If you're not an avid reader or do not work directly with words then you might be surprised by your limited knowledge of vocabulary. However, with constant practice, you can expand your knowledge of words and overall command of language, which includes your critical reasoning capabilities.

1. Dictionary corner

Select the correct definition from the three options.

1: HOLLOW
A. having a space or cavity inside; empty
B. barren or laid waste; devastated
C. to make a hole or opening

2: ACTIVE
A. without anxiety or worry
B. engaged in action; characterized by energetic work, participation
C. boldly assertive and forward; pushy

3: PRODUCT
A. a person or thing produced by or resulting from a process, such as a natural, social, or historical one; result
B. a continuous action, operation, or series of changes taking place in a definite manner
C. a building or group of buildings with facilities for the manufacture of goods

4: SQUANDER
A. to stake or risk money, or anything of value, on the outcome of something involving chance
B. to spend or use (money, time) extravagantly or wastefully
C. to distribute or apportion by measure; allot; dole out

5: FLOWER
A. the blossom of a plant
B. woody plant smaller than a tree, usually having multiple permanent stems branching from or near the ground
C. a fertile and delightful spot or region

6: PLIANT
A. smooth and agreeable to the touch; not hard or coarse
B. a condition, a state, a situation, especially an unfavorable one
C. bending readily, flexible, supple; adaptable

Solutions on p.182 >>>

2. Like for like

Select the correct synonym from the four options.

1: EUPHORIC
A. lively
B. surprised
C. engrossed
D. ecstatic

2: PIOUS
A. legal
B. devout
C. spirited
D. lucky

3: TIRED
A. infirm
B. fatigued
C. dazed
D. downbeat

4: AUTHENTIC
A. ancient
B. vintage
C. genuine
D. lavish

5: SMART
A. intelligent
B. resolute
C. subtle
D. bullish

6: PERCEPTIVE
A. adept
B. insightful
C. assured
D. resourceful

7: KNAVE
A. slayer
B. storyteller
C. rogue
D. bigot

8: CONCUR
A. defeat
B. agree
C. bolster
D. cooperate

9: MELODIOUS
A. sweet
B. harmonic
C. raucous
D. soulful

10: AMPLE
A. ornate
B. thriving
C. plentiful
D. elegant

11: DODGE
A. disguise
B. net
C. provoke
D. evade

12: MELLOW
A. lament
B. soft
C. frigid
D. exhibitionist

13: OPTIMISTIC
A. reliable
B. righteous
C. hopeful
D. bright

3. Find the opposite

Select the correct antonym from the four options.

1: SHARP
A. chubby
B. blunt
C. boring
D. bright

2: CONSENSUS
A. disagreement
B. teamwork
C. dissension
D. permission

3: SURVIVE
A. nonexistent
B. cease
C. extinct
D. suffer

4: WITHSTAND
A. endure
B. survive
C. succumb
D. possess

5: DAINTY
A. coarse
B. petite
C. superior
D. dirty

6: DAMAGE
A. weaken
B. repair
C. medication
D. evolve

7: DECLINE
A. hesitate
B. accept
C. delegate
D. spurn

8: EXPAND
A. amplify
B. revise
C. shorten
D. skinny

9: FRIENDLY
A. affable
B. evil
C. concerned
D. aloof

10: INQUISITIVE
A. curious
B. clever
C. meddling
D. indifferent

Men and women

It is widely believed that men outperform women in overall spatial ability while women outperform men when it comes to verbal reasoning. But if recent studies are anything to go by, it seems that any difference in verbal aptitude according to gender is negligible. What's more, if the verbal reasoning test includes questions that require spatial processing—for example, solving linear syllogisms (Bob is heavier than Bill, and Bill is heavier than John; who is heaviest?)—then men tend to fare better. However, scientists concede that more research is required.

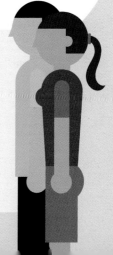

→ Language and intelligence

Fluid intelligence and crystallized intelligence are factors of general intelligence. Fluid intelligence is the ability to find meaning in confusion and solve new problems. Crystallized intelligence refers to the knowledge and skills accumulated over a lifetime and that you apply to do familiar tasks. How does language fit into all this? Well, as a child, you use your fluid intelligence to make sense of the language spoken by your parents and, in turn, learn to communicate with them. During puberty, the rules of grammar, syntax, and all the other nuances of language become crystallized. At this point, the key region of the brain where you imprint new information and skills becomes smaller. It's the reason why learning any language is a lot easier when you are young.

Develop a bilingual brain

It is not impossible to learn a new language in adulthood. In fact we encourage it because, along with taking up a musical instrument, it's one of the best ways to fire up your neurons and keep the brain active. These activities are mentally demanding because they force the brain to process unfamiliar information and make new connections. Learning a foreign language can also help protect the brain against the ravages of aging. Research suggests that people who are bilingual seem to suffer less mental decline from aging than those who speak only one language.

Tips

Here's a rundown of our tips for improving your verbal aptitude:

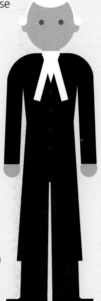

- **Chat with people** from all walks of life. Look beyond family members, friends, and colleagues at work. Be curious. Ask questions. Thoughtful conversations boost your overall cognitive capacity because nanoconnections are happening as you converse. Again, it's another reason why verbal discourse in the form of classroom discussions is a commonly used learning tool.

- **Listen to trained speakers,** such as lawyers or politicians. Concentrate on the thread of their argument. These professionals tend to have a highly developed thinking power based on their mastery over language, and can put across a point effectively.

- **Read more.** Stretch yourself by choosing challenging material. Pick up a classic novel or poem that will introduce you to new words and different styles of writing and original ways of thinking. However, reading in itself is a passive activity, so make a mental note of unfamiliar words and look them up in a dictionary later on. If you are really conscientious, answer the questions "who?", "what?", "where?", "how?", and "why?" at the end of each chapter. As your aptitude for comprehension improves you will naturally begin interacting with the text and this will develop your critical thinking skills.

- **Think out loud!** Verbalizing thoughts not only exercises the left side of your brain but molds abstract concepts, metaphors, and other symbols into more concrete forms.

- **Start a journal.** By writing a daily or weekly journal you will develop your powers of expression, which will have a knock-on effect on your overall verbal aptitude.

- **Complete a daily word puzzle.** Games and exercises such as solving anagrams, rebuses, verbal analogies, and crosswords maintain your verbal aptitude (see pp.130–137). Mix and match the games to give yourself a more holistic workout.

- **Cast a critical eye** over a random horoscope page. It can be any sign and it doesn't matter whether or not you believe in it. Try to extract the main points from the information and summarize them. Be extremely analytical and ask yourself whether the horoscope is revealing anything concrete.

Verbal fluency

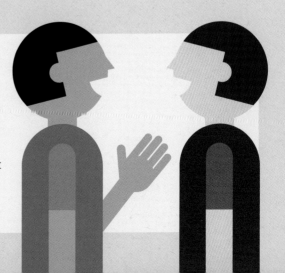

Improving your vocabulary raises your intelligence, plain and simple. The average person's spoken vocabulary is about 1,000 words and the number of words available to feed the brain is over three million. So there's a vast scope for improvement. The broader your vocabulary, the more it will stimulate the brain by firing cell interaction during conversation, reading, and writing. A broad vocabulary gives you an advantage in school, business, and social situations. This is because you are able to think about more complex things precisely. Verbal fluency will give you the double advantage of thinking more quickly under pressure and talking more composedly under duress.

A workout with words

Here is a selection of fun exercises to help sharpen your verbal aptitude. They are designed to combine your visual sense with your verbal reasoning skills.

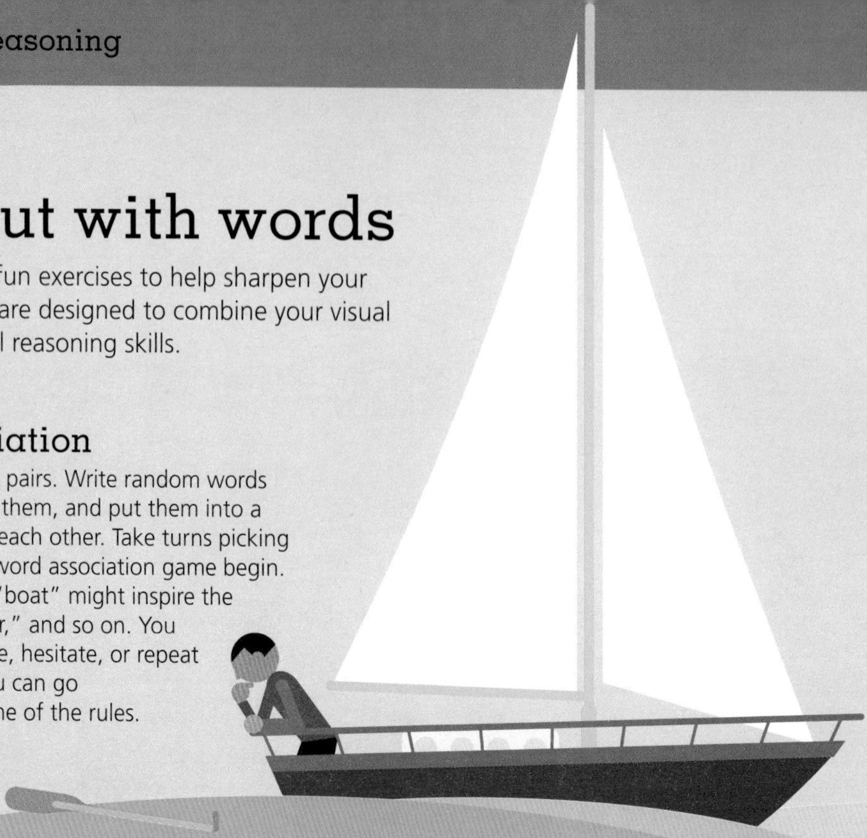

4. Word association

This is a game to play in pairs. Write random words on scraps of paper, fold them, and put them into a box. Sit down and face each other. Take turns picking out a word and let the word association game begin. For example, the word "boat" might inspire the word "sail," "sea," "oar," and so on. You are not allowed to pause, hesitate, or repeat a word. See how far you can go until someone breaks one of the rules.

5. Colored words

In the fastest time possible, say aloud the color the word is printed in, trying not to read the word. This exercise works both hemispheres of the brain, with neurons zapping between the verbal and visual sites as you try to manage your attention, inhibiting one response in order to say something else.

seconds

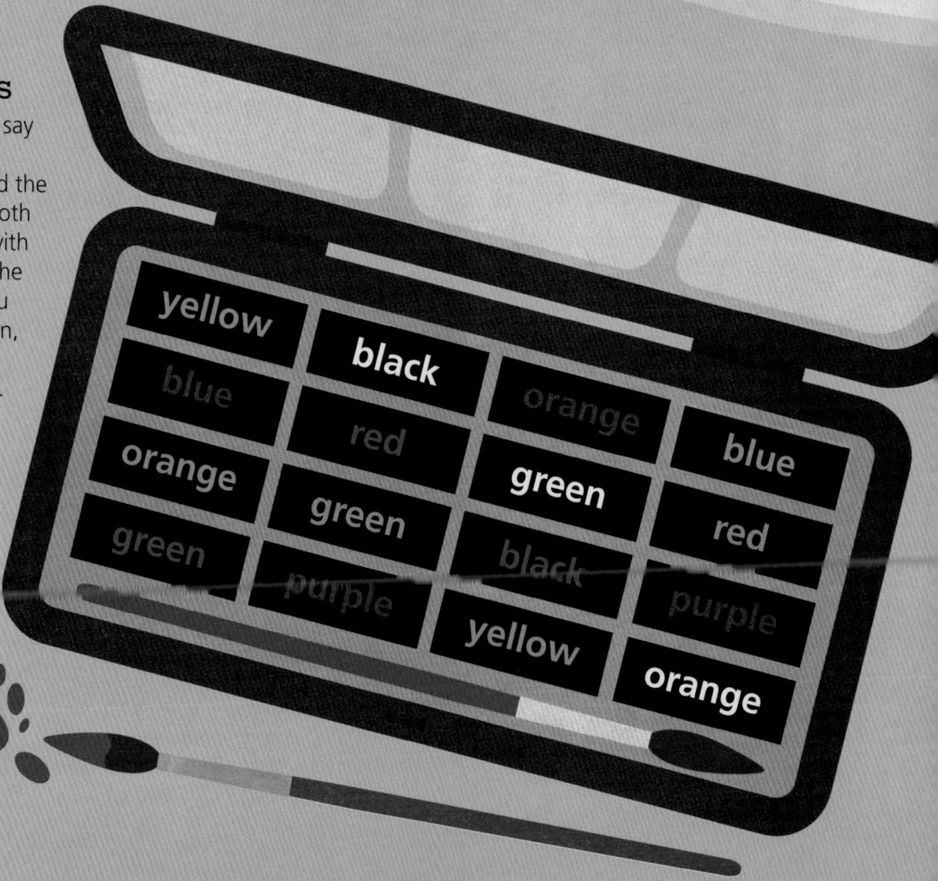

yellow   black   orange   blue

blue   red   green   red

orange   green   black   purple

green   purple   yellow   orange

6. Scrambled sentences

Unscramble the following list of words to make a normal sentence. Notice how your eyes keep stalling because the brain cannot make sense of the words, which disrupts your natural reading rhythm. This is a harder exercise than you might think.

A: a teacher Margaret school is strict

B: circulation improves to exercise Physical brain blood the

C: brain of billion 100 consists Your about neurons

D: exercise is brain-training a Sudoku good

E: words average The reading 200–250 speed is minute a

F: read You are you what

G: reading experience eyes By another life through you by vicariously the of

H: reasoning use find assess candidate verbal out verbal tests well how a can logic to Interviewers

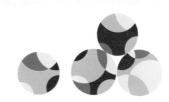

Solution on p.182

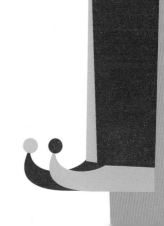

7. The word ladder

Use association to get from the first object to the last. This is more demanding than game 4 because you have to use your verbal aptitude to get to a fixed destination.

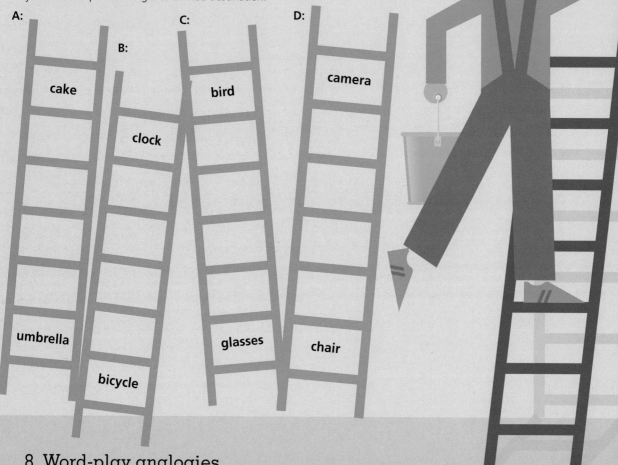

A:
- cake
- umbrella

B:
- clock
- bicycle

C:
- bird
- glasses

D:
- camera
- chair

8. Word-play analogies

Identify the correct analogy that would make each statement true.

A: *Come* is to *go* as *arrival* is to ...	B: *Arm* is to *hand* as *leg* is to ...	C: *Right* is to *left* as *below* is to ...	D: *Rose* is to *flower* as *dog* is to ...
terminus	foot	ground	cat
airport	toe	above	human
depot	ankle	ceiling	animal
departure	sole	cellar	puppy

9. Student lodgings

A: Andrew, Bruce, Caroline, David, Emma, Fiona, George, and Harriet are all friends who met at college. As students, they lived together in different groups. The diagram below shows how they were grouped.

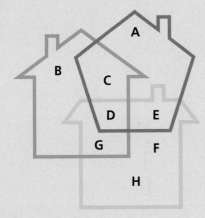

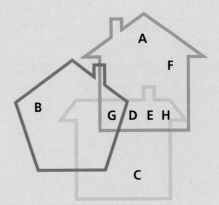

1. Which person/s lived in all three houses?

2. Which person/s lived in house 1 (green) and house 2 (blue) but not in house 3 (red)?

3. Which person/s lived in house 1 (green) for the entire year?

4. Which person/s moved from house 1 (green) to house 3 (red)?

5. Which person/s remained in house 2 (blue) all year?

6. Which person/s lived in all three houses?

7. Who is the only person Bruce lived with this year?

8. Which house held the most people?

C: People moved once more in the final year. The diagram below shows how they were grouped.

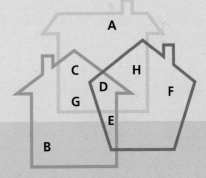

B: The following year people moved into different houses. The next diagram (above, right) shows how they were grouped.

E: *Love* is to *hate*
as *heat* is to ...
warmth
ice
burning
cold

9. Which person/s lived in all three houses?

10. Which person/s lived in house 2 (blue) and house 3 (red) but not in house 1 (green)?

11. Which person/s has Andrew lived with during all three years?

12. Which person/s has Andrew never lived with?

Solutions on p.182 »»

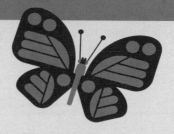

10. Odd one out
Which object is the odd one out?

A:
Car
Bus
Train
Truck

B:
Bonnet
Fez
Cap
Stocking

C:
Tiger
Cheetah
Leopard
Jaguar

D:
Rock
Log
Boulder
Pebble

E:
Tomato
Carrot
Cabbage
Spinach

F:
Clavichord
Spinet
Harpsichord
Clarion

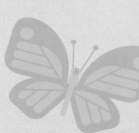

11. Spot the errors!
It's easy today. Usually, when writing, you use a word processing program on a computer, equipped with spellchecker software, which automatically corrects any misspelled words, or flags them with a red squiggle. However, spotting a spelling error is harder than you might think. This is because you see words as a complete pattern rather than the sum of letter parts. To put it another way, you tend to recognize words even if some of the units may not be correct. Another reason for this is that you rely on contextual information to help recognize individual words during ordinary reading.

Read the following passage and try to pick out all the mistakes.

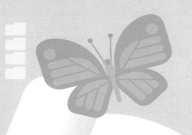

Only last night, I arguued with my fiend about the correct speling of a word: I said the correct spelling was "commited" while my friend insisted that it's "comitted." Actually I am surprised that people can make so many spelling errors. Often when you ponit out people's mistakes they feel criticized. Of coarse, the last thing I want to do is offend anybody; I just think it is good for ones personal developement to improve there spelling. I've also found that if you point out people's spelling errors some people just get embarrassed, or became really defensive. I am realy happy to report that the collage I go to is implimenting measures to tackle bad spelling; they are drawering up classes to teach students hoe to asess what they read correctly. I think its worng for any teacher to ignore a student's bad spelling, and not prapare then adequately to go out into the wider world. We should, however, remembar that bad spelling and bad thinking are completly seperate issues. Just because your a bad speller doesn't make you dum. All it means is that you need to work harder to improve your spelling. It will really make a big differance when you start sending you're CV to employers as to weather or not you get an interview.

12. Fill in the blanks

Choose the correct word from the list to complete the sentences A–G.

1. Trouncing
2. Fireman
3. Bombarding
4. Extend
5. Expand
6. Scientist
7. Mesmerizing

A: Jasper, our pet dog, started barking when he saw the .... break the lock and climb in through the window. Jasper had locked all of us out.

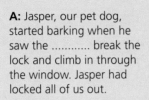

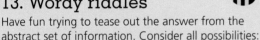

B: The poet had an elegant voice. She was .... us with her beautifully written verses.

C: If "Beauty is in the eye of the beholder" then why do magazines keep ...... us with retouched images?

D: It's a fact that roosters cannot crow if they cannot .... their necks.

E: We've been telling Jim to........... his horizons.

F: The team won by .... the opposition.

G: When Ian started out as a .... he wore his lab coat with the buttons done up to his neck.

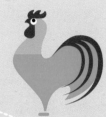

13. Wordy riddles

Have fun trying to tease out the answer from the abstract set of information. Consider all possibilities:

A: I can be heard but am never seen.
Once I come out I never go back in.
If you recognize me you'll know
where I've come from. What am I?

B: If there are three cups of sugar and you take one away, how many do you have?

C: A prisoner was found guilty and was due to be sentenced. The judge decided to test his verbal reasoning powers and said to him, "You may make a statement. If it is true, I'll sentence you to 4 years in prison. If it is false, I'll sentence you to 6 years in prison." After the prisoner had thought for a bit and made his statement, the judge decided to let him go free. What did the prisoner say?

D: All things I devour,
birds, beasts, trees, and flowers;
I gnaw through iron, and I bite
through steel;
I grind hard stones to meal;
I slay kings, I lay waste
to towns,
I even bring high mountains down.
What am I?

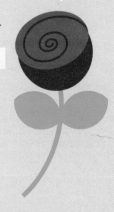

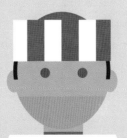

Solutions on pp.182–3 »»

Reading comprehension

Reading comprehension is an essential part of language development. The ability to understand and interact with the text works your brain in multiple ways, honing your perception, reason, problem solving, and other cognitive faculties. It is a fundamental skill to which you are introduced as a child, develop as a student, and then apply in your career as well as your everyday life. A typical reading comprehension assessment usually involves answering a series of questions relating to a given passage of writing. The exercise tests your ability to draw logical inferences from simple life situations. Your answers indicate how well you interpret the material.

An eye for reading

Comprehension requires good reading, which depends on your ability to recognize words rapidly and effortlessly. This is where your eyes play a major role since the information is transferred via the visual pathways. The average reading rate for a Roman-character-based language is 200–220 words per minute. Anything less will interfere with your ability to decode the meaning because you will be putting more effort into reading individual words or sentences than trying to understand the idea being expressed.

14. Summer job

Read the passage and give your answer to each question as either "true," "false," or "cannot say."

Post offices find it beneficial to employ students over their vacations. Permanent members of the staff often wish to take their own vacations during this period. Furthermore, it is not uncommon for post offices to experience peak workloads during the holiday period and so require extra staff. Holiday employment also attracts students who may wish to return as qualified recruits to post offices once they have completed their education. Ensuring that the students learn as much as possible about the post office encourages interest in working on a permanent basis. Post offices pay students at a fixed rate without the usual right to benefits.

Statement A—It is possible that permanent staff who are on vacation can have their work carried out by students.

Statement B—Students employed over their vacation period given the same paid vacation benefit as permanent staff.

Statement C—Students are subject to the post office's standard disciplinary and grievance procedures.

Common strategies to tackle reading comprehension:

• Begin with a thorough reading to get the general gist without stopping in midflow.
• Summarize what you read.
• Track what you are reading to make sure that it makes sense throughout.
• Highlight salient points.
• Anticipate and predict so that you interact with text.

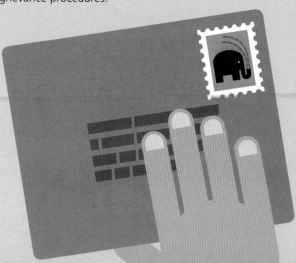

15. The sounds in my life

Read the passage and based on your understanding of it, check the box that correctly completes each sentence.

I was walking along the street of my village when I heard the siren of a fire engine sounding in the distance. As I turned, I saw two other people turning to look in the same direction.

The sound of any passing emergency vehicle is an instant attention-grabber in my village.

In contrast, people living in a city are exposed to so many sounds that they become desensitized and don't really pay much attention when they hear an emergency vehicle in the distance.

I was the same when I used to work in the city many years ago. I hardly ever noticed any sounds while sitting at my desk, even when the window was wide open.

It's very different at home here in the village. If I'm in bed, the sound of an aircraft flying high over the house can wake me up.

It's the quieter sounds that affect me the most. Sometimes, in the middle of the night, I can hear scratching noises downstairs. I also hear little creaking noises, which my imagination turns into footsteps. This has been going on for the last 25 years. I'm not sure why I never hear these sounds during the day.

I have a good idea of sounds I like and sounds that I don't. I no longer like the sound of a dog barking. It never used to bother me but now it reminds me of the time I got bitten and whenever I hear the sound, my palms begin to sweat and my body tenses up.

The sound of the keys of my typewriter hitting the paper is lovely. I often write so that I can listen to the sound my typewriter makes.

1. The sound of a fire engine in the village makes people …
A: think of a fire
B: look at each other
C: pay attention to it
D: stop crossing the street

2. People in the city …
A: don't care about emergencies
B: are used to sirens
C: are attracted by sounds
D: don't hear loud noises

3. The writer …
A: sleeps next to the window
B: isn't sure what causes the noises at night
C: believes in ghosts
D: is interested in aircraft

4. The writer relates to sounds at night by …
A: imagining sounds that do not exist
B: exaggerating quiet sounds
C: imagining the sound of doors shutting
D: refusing to acknowledge them

5. The writer dislikes the sound of a dog's bark because …
A: it doesn't affect her
B: it reminds her of happier times
C: it makes her feel tense
D: it is too loud

6. The writer enjoys the sound of …
A: a coin dropping on the pavement
B: her typewriter when she's typing
C: anything that attracts her attention
D: footsteps

7. The writer thinks the sounds in her life are …
A: making her miserable
B: louder now because she's more attuned to them
C: a general mixture of good and bad
D: a lot better at night because they affect her the most

Solutions on p.183 »»

→ Words and pictures

Historians have traced the art of storytelling, which uses a sequence of pictures, all the way back to the earliest human civilizations. However, the art form that combines words and pictures evolved much later on. For example, it wasn't until the American comic strip format arrived in the early 20th century that devices such as the word balloon for speech, the symbol of the flashing light bulb above a character's head to indicate a bright idea, and specific typographical symbols to represent cursing were introduced. The first comic books were anthologies collected from newspapers, which ran adventure stories such as *Buck Rogers*, *Tarzan*, *The Phantom*, and *The Adventures of TinTin* in comic strip format. The late Will Eisner, a famous cartoonist, called them "sequential art" as opposed to "comic strips."

Over the years many educational institutions have used comic strip narratives to develop verbal reasoning and comprehension skills. We respond more positively to the combination of words and pictures. In a world overloaded with visual material we have become more image-savvy and, therefore, comic strips offer a fun and effective way to boost literacy. You can do a fun exercise by cutting up the comic strips into individual cells, shuffling them, and then trying to put them back together. You might even find an alternative way to piece the cells to construct a different story altogether!

Solution on p.183 »»

16. Dog's day out

We've removed the text from the speech bubbles in the comic strip and listed it below. Using the visual cues, try to put the correct text into the correct bubble so that the dialogue makes sense.

- *It's good to have a city break!*
- *Mad mutt!*
- *Behave yourself Orca.*
- *Oh, the usual.*
- *Woof!*
- *LATER...*
- *Mineral water please, no ice.*
- *Did you have a good day?*
- *Here we go ...*
- *SOON ...*
- *Woof!*
- *I'm off to school ... be a good dog today!*
- *Crazy dog!*
- *ONE MORNING ...*
- *I'll try ... but I have a short memory.*
- *About time too ...*
- *LATER STILL ...*
- *As if I'd be anything else.*

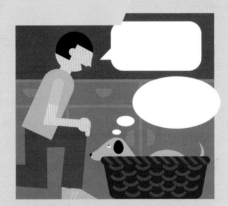
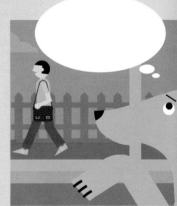
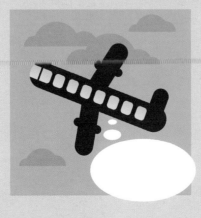
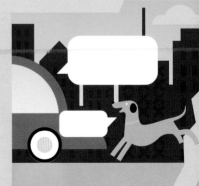

Verbal or visual?

A recent psychology study, using functional magnetic resonance imaging (fMRI) technology to scan the brain, revealed that those who regard themselves to be visual learners, as opposed to verbal learners, have a natural tendency to convert linguistically presented information into a visual mental representation. The more strongly an individual relied on the visual cognitive style, the more that individual activated the visual cortex when presented with any reading matter.

According to the study, the opposite also appears to be the case. Those participants who considered themselves verbal learners were found under fMRI to have brain activity in the region associated with language cognition when faced with a picture (see p.125), suggesting they have a tendency to convert pictorial information into linguistic representations.

Future research based on these findings may be able to determine whether cognitive styles are something one is predisposed to or can learn. Depending on the flexibility with which one can adopt a style, educators could cater to one style over another to improve learning.

It has long been thought that propensities for visual or verbal learning styles influence how children acquire knowledge successfully and how adults reason in everyday life.

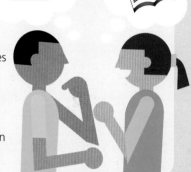

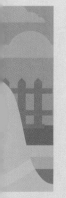
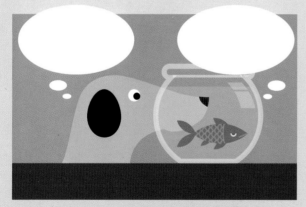
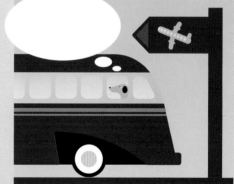
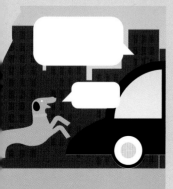
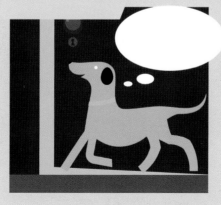
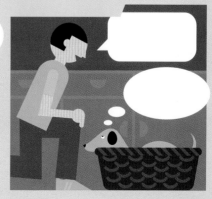

Build a story

Storytelling is an ancient oral art that demonstrates the power of words to express thoughts, ideas, and feelings. We have relied upon it for spreading news, imparting wisdom, and learning the cultural history of others and ourselves. Storytelling is a commonly used tool for making connections with people of all ages and races.

It is also a very powerful tool that develops and strengthens skills in the language areas of semantics (meaning of words), syntax (formation of words), phonology (speech sounds), and so on. Storytelling uses language artistically to develop all of the critical components involved in the communication process. Storytelling improves listening skills, enhances verbal expression, increases comprehension, creates mental images, and stimulates verbal reasoning. It is the most holistic way to hone your verbal aptitude.

Taking our cue from this, we will end this chapter with two exercises that will test your creative writing skills.

17. A mini-adventure

Write a paragraph that is no longer than 60 words, referring to the 6 objects below in no particular order.

Here are your 6 objects:

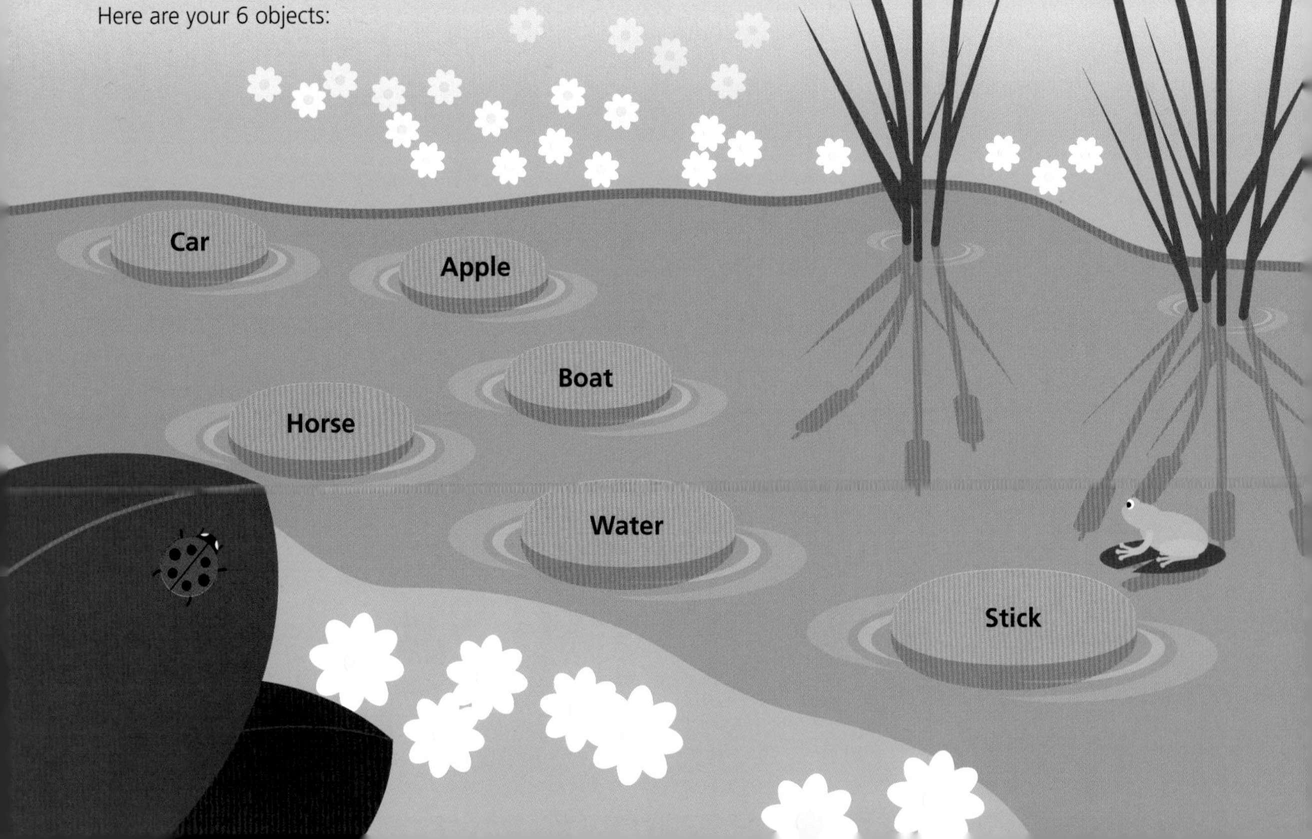

Car

Apple

Boat

Horse

Water

Stick

18. The main feature

This is an extension of the first exercise. This time we have provided you with a larger array of objects. They have been separated into 3 groups. Your aim is to write a 250-word story each time, using the objects from the following groups:

A: Group 1
B: Group 2
C: Group 3
D: Groups 1+3
E: Groups 2+3

Group 3

Group 1

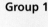

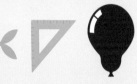
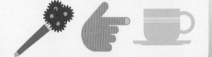

Group 2

Did you know?

Human beings have a natural tendency to make stories out of everything. It is part of a larger desire and need to put ourselves in another person's shoes—to be able to empathize. It is crucial to social interaction and communal living. Psychologists call this Theory of Mind. A classic 1944 study clearly demonstrated this tendency. The psychologists showed people an animation of a pair of triangles and a circle moving around a square and asked the participants what was happening. The subjects described the scene as if the shapes had intentions and motivations—for example,

"The circle is chasing the triangles." Many studies since then have confirmed the human predilection to make characters and narratives out of whatever we see in the world around us. Some psychologists believe that the imaginary world of a story may serve as a proving ground for vital social skills.

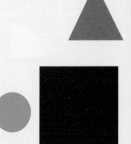

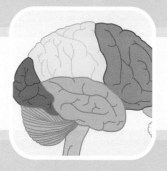

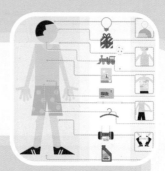

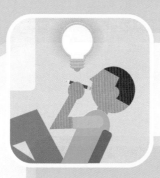

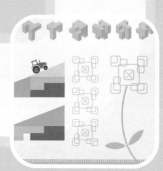

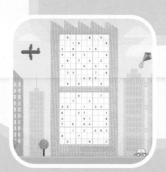

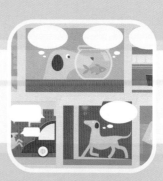

Chapter 7

The mind-body connection

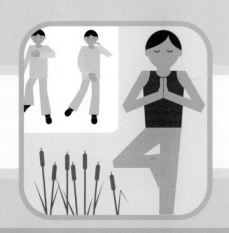

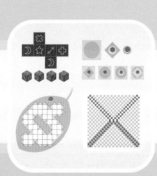

Healthy body, sturdy mind

We all need some physical exercise to stay in shape. Nobody would disagree with that. But how does the brain feature in all this? Well, there's a famous Latin saying from ancient Roman times: "*mens sana in corpore sano*," meaning "a healthy mind in a healthy body." It seems that the Romans were onto something here because, while we've known for a long time that physical exercise can maintain general health and well-being, more research findings are indicating that exercise may also be one of the best ways to preserve brain health.

Actually, even if successive scientific studies hadn't revealed this, it would be astonishing if this were *not* the case. Any physical activity, even a five-minute jog in place at the start of each day, raises our heart rate, which in turn increases blood flow throughout the body—including the brain. The positive effects of physical exercise are more noticeable the older you get. People in their 50s who exercise regularly generally have better memories and greater concentration spans than those who lead sedentary lives. What's more, those people who keep physically active into their 60s reduce the likelihood of suffering mental decline because some age-related cognitive diseases result from physical inactivity, as well as a lack of mental stimulation.

What is aerobic exercise?

It's any physical activity, such as walking, jogging, or dancing, that increases the heart rate to 60–80 percent of its maximum capacity for a period of 15 minutes or longer. This allows the lungs to draw in more oxygen, which the heart pumps through the vascular system. You should be able to engage in a conversation while doing aerobic exercise. If you haven't exercised in a while, we advise you to have a thorough physical checkup before you begin any exercise program.

How much exercise?

Guidelines published by the World Health Organization (WHO) recommends at least 30 minutes of moderate-intensity physical exercise, such as a gentle jog, per day. However, the majority of health professionals agree that most people can reap greater health benefits by engaging in activity that's either more intense for a shorter burst of time, or less strenuous but carried out over a longer period. You could also add stretching for flexibility, and resistance exercises called "calisthenics" to improve muscle strength and tone.

Let's assess your exercise history—past and present

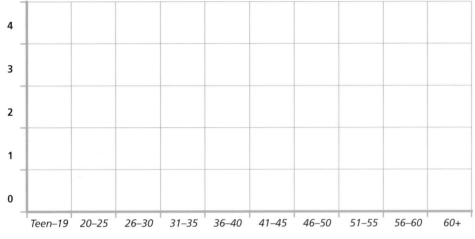

	Teen–19	20–25	26–30	31–35	36–40	41–45	46–50	51–55	56–60	60+	
4											Exercise four times a week +
3											Exercise three times a week
2											Exercise twice a week
1											Exercise once a week
0											No exercise

Plot the graph by giving yourself a rating between 0 and 4 to assess how much physical exercise you do (30 minutes +), or have done in the past. For example, if you played tennis twice a week as a teenager, put a 2 in that box. If you went jogging once a week, write in 1. If you don't do any exercise at the moment, put 0 in the appropriate box. Complete the relevant age sections. How do your scores compare over the different periods of your life? Many people tend to show a decline in their level of physical activity with age, but you should try to keep exercising to maintain your physical and cognitive health.

How exercise works the brain

Any form of aerobic exercise is the best way to improve blood circulation to the brain. The increased blood flow helps the frontal lobes, in particular (see p.14). The frontal lobes control emotional activity and play a key role in mental sharpness. It is the region you use to process thoughts to make decisions, pay attention, show initiative, find humor in things, and so on. Unfortunately, this is also the part of the brain that feels the brunt of the aging process, making people forgetful, slow on the uptake, and less verbally fluent as they get older.

Exercise combats this decline by:
1. Generating a chemical called BDNF (brain-derived neurotrophic factor), which acts a bit like fertilizer for the brain's existing neurons, and encourages the growth of new neurons and synapses.

2. Increasing the amount of serotonin in the brain—this brain chemical helps cells multiply and induces positive moods.

3. Causing new tiny blood vessels called capillaries to sprout and nourish brain cells that might otherwise wilt from the aging process.

4. Boosting the growth of neural stem cells. Studies involving mice exercised on treadmills for an hour a day against mice that were left sedentary showed that the mice that were exercised had twice the number of cells, making them smarter.

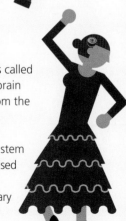

The physical recharge

It's difficult to sustain energy levels through the course of an entire working day. At some point fatigue might set in, or you might feel as if your brain can no longer think clearly. When the feeling strikes, a lot of people drink coffee or reach for a chocolate bar, relying on the caffeine or sugar spike to bring energy levels back up. But this is both unhealthy and a short-term solution. An alternative way to boost energy is by engaging in a simple physical activity for a few minutes, which improves blood circulation and instantly makes you more alert. Here are some of the best ways to give yourself a physical charge.

Warmups

"Warming up" before playing any physical sport is normal. Athletes warm up not just to prepare physically, but also to focus their mind and access "muscle memory." By warming up in tennis, for example, the body and mind synchronize to remember the different strokes and actions required for a game. This brain-muscle synergy decreases the likelihood of a bad performance or injury. Another important benefit of warming up is that it helps you relax and hone concentration.

1. Take a simple walk ... or climb the stairs

A gentle walk is a good pickup because it increases blood circulation and the amount of oxygen and glucose that reach your brain. Walking is not strenuous, so your leg muscles don't take up extra oxygen and glucose, as they do during other forms of exercise. Maybe this is why walking can "clear your head." If you don't have the time for a stroll, then climb some stairs. This gets your heart rate up quicker and boosts blood circulation—a perfect pickup prior to entering a meeting room or taking an examination.

2. Cross crawl warmup

1. Walk or jog on the spot.
2. Lift your left knee to your right elbow, then repeat for a count of 5–10.
3. Now lift your right knee to your left elbow and repeat the movement.
4. Keep a steady rhythm for a minute.

The cross crawl is a simple and powerful energy technique to promote access to both the right and left-brain hemispheres. The crossing over of energy helps you feel more balanced, think more clearly, and improves coordination.

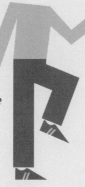

3. Side-to-side warmup

1. Raise left arm and right leg and sway slightly to the left.
2. Then return to neutral position. Change over by raising right arm and left leg and sway to the right.
3. Repeat movement for one minute, keeping steady rhythm without straining too much.

5. Massaging the K-27 points

Place fingers on your collarbone. Slide them inward toward the center and find the bumps where they stop. Move your fingers down about an inch. Most people have a slight indent here that their fingers will drop into—these are the K-27 points. Cross your hands if you wish; tap and/or massage the K-27 points while breathing in through your nose and out through your mouth. Continue for about 20 seconds. If you're using one hand, tap on both points with thumb and fingers.

When you massage the K-27 points on a regular basis, you should experience a slight energy surge, clearer thinking, and improved vision.

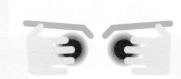

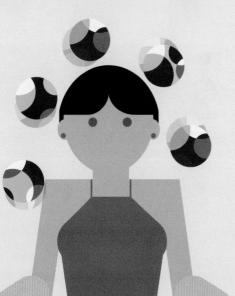

4. Juggle

Juggling may seem faintly ludicrous, but don't underestimate this dexterous pursuit as a way to help take your mind off the stresses of the daily grind. It will help improve hand-eye coordination and, according to one university study, may also boost your brainpower.

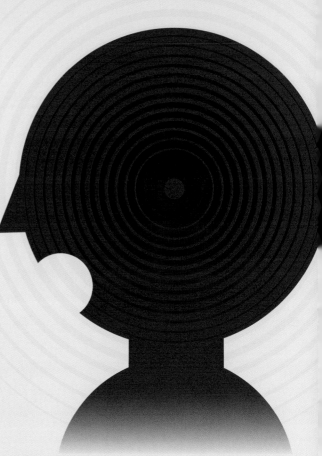

Stress factor

Stress builds up when a person becomes overwhelmed by the pressures of life and feels unable to cope. The key word here is "feel," because stress is about the perception of the demands on the mind, which has a knock-on effect on physical well-being. Stress weakens powers of creativity and memory recall. Stress isn't all bad—everyone needs to experience moderate levels to maintain focus and feel stimulated—but when it becomes excessive and unmanageable its effect is counterproductive and, potentially, detrimental to our health. Chemicals called glutamates are pumped into the brain, which can be harmful. A person becomes frazzled by too many demands, loses self-confidence, and ends up feeling flustered, and, as a result, may become forgetful, misplace things, misinterpret conversations, snap at others, and so on. Excessive stress causes both brain and body to become inefficient.

Mind-body checklist

Before we introduce you to a gentle de-stressing routine, complete this checklist, checking the boxes that best describe your current physical state.

	Very tense	Quite tense	Quite relaxed	Very relaxed
Face				
Forehead				
Back of neck				
Shoulders				
Chest				
Back				
Stomach				
Groin				
Buttocks				
Legs				
Feet				
Arms				
Hands				

The physical stress-buster

If you found that the majority of your checks fell in the "very tense" or "quite tense" box, then you need to find a way to regulate your stress levels. Many people use a popular technique called Progressive Muscle Relaxation (PMR). PMR is about exaggerating the feeling of tension to help the mind and body wind down. You tense each muscle group of the body in turn until it starts to hurt—for about 20 seconds—and then let go. Blood rushes to the area, which creates a warm sensation, and the tension should then flow away, leaving a state of total calm. PMR can work as a sleep aid as well.

The PMR program

Sit on a chair, with your back straight and both feet flat on the ground.
Do the exercises in the following order: (remember to tense for 20 seconds):

1.	Right hand and forearm	make a fist, hold, then release
2.	Right upper arm	bend the arm and "flex the bicep," then release
3.	Left hand and forearm	make a fist, hold, then release
4.	Left upper arm	bend the arm and "flex the bicep," then release
5.	Forehead	raise your eyebrows, then relax your face
6.	Face	squeeze the eyes, then relax; clench your teeth and pull the corners of the mouth back, then relax
7.	Shoulders and neck	lock your hands behind your neck and gently push your head back against this resistance (the head does not alter its position); raise your shoulders and press your head back against their resistance (horizontally, unlike when you look up); let your shoulders hang, relax
8.	Chest and back	inhale deeply and hold your breath, puffing out your chest at the same time as letting your shoulders hang, then breathe normally
9.	Belly	tighten the abdominal muscles (or draw in the belly), then release
10.	Right thigh	push the right foot forward using the floor as resistance (just enough so the chair doesn't rock back), then release
11.	Right calf	lift up the right heel, then release
12.	Right foot	crook the toes, then release
13.	Left thigh	push the left foot forward using the floor as resistance (just enough so the chair doesn't rock back), then release
14.	Left calf	lift up the left heel, then release
15.	Left foot	crook the toes, then release

Exercise the Eastern way

For thousands of years in the East, people have harnessed a whole range of techniques to seek harmony between mind, body, and spirit. Although traditionally, Western medicine has been sceptical of Eastern therapies, such as Zen, T'ai Chi, and yoga, increasing evidence from scientific studies, especially using brain scanning techniques, indicates that the ancient Eastern monks really knew ways of lowering blood pressure, slowing respiration, releasing muscle tension, and decluttering the mind. In today's fast-paced world, people are exposed to greater pressures. The body usually reacts by releasing stress-response hormones such as cortisol, which circulates the system and inadvertently blocks the formation of new neurons in the hippocampus. We now know that any type of meditative exercise helps the body regulate stress hormone levels.

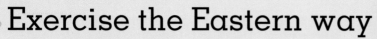
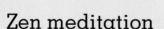

Zen meditation

Zen meditation is a practice that lies at the core of Zen belief. The purpose is to focus the mind—sometimes through using a mantra, a sound, or the breath—and promote a state of absolute calm. Through sitting still and honing the attention on a simple chant, the meditator unclutters all the bric-a-brac he or she stores in the head, namely negative thoughts, emotions, and sensations. This state of mind is often called "mindfulness."

About 10 million people meditate every day in the West and while there are many different techniques, the primary objective is to become aware of the stream of thoughts, allowing them to arise and pass away without interference. Empirical evidence suggests that Zen meditation helps alleviate the symptoms of depression and also improves quality of sleep.

Enter the meditative state

It is important to adopt a good posture whether you choose to sit or stand, always keeping the back upright. The aim is to clear the mind of all distractions and reach a state of "no mind" or "nonthinking." To achieve this you have to pay attention to the sensory experience, rather than to your thoughts about the sensory experience, or anything else for that matter. For example, if you suddenly hear a noise, you just listen to it rather than think about it. As soon as you enter the meditative state, your brainwave patterns should shift from the right frontal cortex to the calmer left frontal cortex. This decreases the negative effects of stress, mild depression, and anxiety.

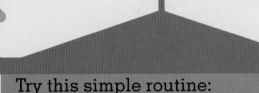

Try this simple routine:

1. Find a quiet spot.

2. Sit on a chair, stool, or cushion with your back straight and unsupported.

3. Inhale and exhale slowly through your nose.

4. Close your eyes and relax your body (but keep your back relatively straight).

5. Listen to your breathing; lose yourself in the rhythm of the breath.

6. Start to hum or say "om" with each breath, keeping the sound constant; think about the vibration of the hum. Alternatively, repeat a chant or phrase such as "don't worry, be happy."

7. Whisper or say the word quietly in your mind.

8. Keep this going for 5 minutes. How do you feel now?

Focus your mind

You can also meditate by focusing your mind on an object, such as a candle flame. By focusing all your energies on a single object, you are blocking out all the other stimuli that bring sensations, emotions, thoughts, daydreams, and impressions. In other words, your mind ceases to swing from branch to branch and comes to a tranquil state, which naturally destresses your entire system.

T'ai Chi

T'ai Chi is an ancient martial art that combines physical exercise with mental exercise. The emphasis on movement helps expand the mind and channel the body's energy. Focusing the mind on the slow movements creates a state of mental calm and clarity. Medical studies support its effectiveness as a form of therapy for managing stress. These studies conclude that practicing T'ai Chi regularly will help you relax, stay focused, and be more productive in life.

How does T'ai Chi work?

T'ai Chi practitioners believe that the intense concentration and the slow movements improve the flow of energy throughout the body. They consider this to be positive energy, as opposed to the negative energy induced by anger, for example, which is damaging to health.

Try this simple test:

1. Sit down and think of a time when you were frustrated or angry about something. It could be an instance when a reckless driver cut into your lane, or a time when someone was being unreasonable to you at your workplace.

2. Recall what happened, the people involved—you will feel the anger and resentment returning.

3. Notice how this makes your body tense up and how your breathing rate increases.

Dredging up an unpleasant memory from the past affects your body. Now, try this:

1. Stand upright, relax your shoulders.

2. Raise your hand in front of you and begin slowly rotating your wrist clockwise, concentrating on the movement as well as your breathing. Do this for a minute.

3. The tension should slowly abate and your breathing slow down.

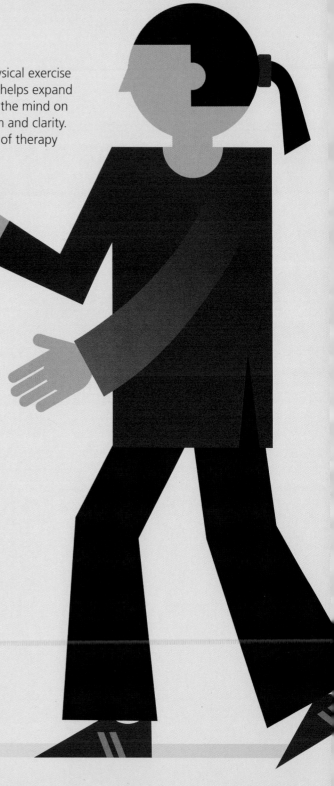

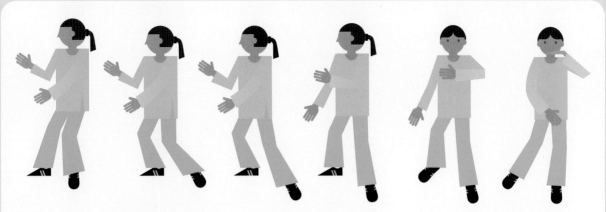

A sequence of T'ai Chi moves

The benefits of practicing T'ai Chi are unlimited. Clinical studies in the US report improved balance and peace of mind after only eight weeks of a very simple set of movements taken from a T'ai Chi routine. T'ai Chi can be used as a preventive health measure, to maintain good health, and/or to help with managing a specific ailment. It can also improve internal circulation. Studies suggest that patients who suffer from neurological diseases, such as Parkinson's or Alzheimer's, might also benefit from practicing T'ai Chi on a regular basis.

Acupuncture and the brain

Acupuncture is an ancient Chinese treatment for many illnesses, in which a practitioner inserts fine needles in defined points of a patient's body through which "Qi," the vital energy, flows. There are more than 1,500 "acupoints" throughout the body. Acupuncture works by deactivating, or "quieting down," key regions of the brain, and is used to alleviate acute mood states, pain, and cravings. The science behind this is far from understood, and clinical trials into acupuncture remain inconclusive. However, several studies involving volunteers who were monitored using fMRI brain scans revealed that blood flow decreased in certain areas of their brain within seconds of undergoing an acupuncture session. Other studies have found acupuncture to be helpful in treating depression, eating disorders, addictions, and pain, although critics believe that the positive results could easily be a result of the placebo effect. There is general agreement that acupuncture is safe when administered by a qualified practitioner using sterile needles. However, many physicians reject the treatment altogether because the idea of the "Qi" and its various pathways does not reconcile with modern biomedical knowledge.

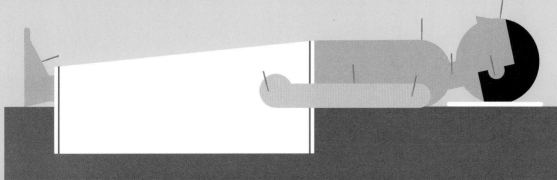

Yoga

Yoga is an ancient practice that originated in India and is more than 5,000 years old. Similar to T'ai Chi, it combines breathing exercises with physical postures and meditation. However, whereas T'ai Chi is classified as a soft martial art, asking you to focus energy on the elegance of motion, yoga is more like a conventional body workout. It's about holding specific postures and controlling breathing. Yoga is thought to calm the nervous system and balance the body and mind. Some of its practitioners claim that yoga can prevent certain maladies by keeping the energy pathways open and life-energy flowing.

The popularity of yoga has grown throughout the world. Yoga has been used to lower blood pressure, reduce stress, and improve coordination, flexibility, concentration, sleep, and digestion. One study has found that doing yoga regularly elevates brain gamma-aminobutyric acid levels (GABA)—an amino acid that plays an important role in regulating neuronal excitability throughout the nervous system. It recommends that the practice of yoga be explored as a possible treatment for depression and anxiety disorders associated with low GABA levels.

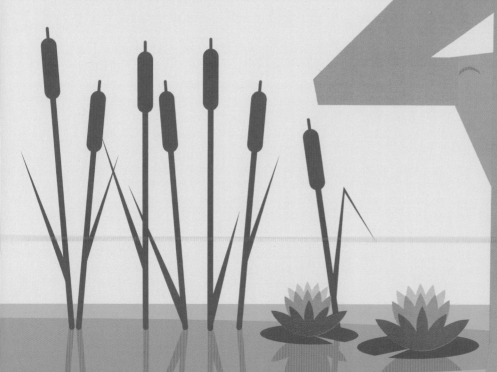

Yoga poses

Here are three basic poses to try. If you haven't exercised in a while, you might need to ease yourself slowly to increase body flexibility. We advise that you start with a medical checkup or consult a yoga practitioner. The poses are arranged in the approximate order of difficulty.

Mountain pose

This pose promotes confidence and a positive mental state, as well as improving posture and circulation.

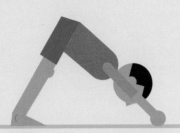

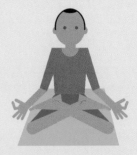

• Stand upright with your feet together. Fan out your toes and push your feet against the floor as if to stretch them.

• Feel the thigh muscles stretch upward and your kneecaps rise a little.

• Keep your body weight evenly distributed. Draw in your abdomen and maintain a high chest so that you take deep, even breaths. Keep your arms at your sides.

Downward dog

An all-round energizer that improves circulation and concentration.

• Inhale, come down on all fours, tucking your toes under.

• Exhale, drawing your abdomen toward your spine and lifting your pelvis to form an inverted "V," with your body in the position illustrated.

• Keep your arms and legs straight (if possible) and turn your armpits to face each other.

• Push your buttocks up and stretch back and down with your heels, with your breathing even and smooth. Remain in the pose for 20 seconds.

Lotus

This is one of the most popular meditative postures. It promotes balance and harmony by calming the mind.

• Sit in a cross-legged position with the soles of your feet turned upward and heels as close to your abdomen as possible. Keep your spine straight.

• Rest your hands on your knees, palms up. Hold as long as you wish.

• Keep the head erect and the eyes closed during this posture.

Brain training with meditation

Neurologists have discovered that during meditative exercises, such as yoga and T'ai Chi, brainwave patterns change and neuronal firing patterns synchronize. The left prefrontal cortex, an area just behind the left side of the forehead, has been identified as the place where brain activity associated with meditation is especially intense. MRI scans carried out on Tibetan monks found that meditating actually increases the thickness of the prefrontal cortex, which is involved in attention and sensory processing. This is sound proof that people who mediate regularly actually alter their brain anatomy. Consistant meditators also develop a remarkable ability to cultivate positive emotions, retain emotional stability, and engage in mindful behavior.

Sleep and the brain

There is nothing as refreshing as a good night's sleep. You wake up feeling revitalized and ready to face the day's challenges. This is because during sleep, growth hormones are released to heal damaged tissue, including brain tissue. Sleep also oils the cogs of the cognitive system by "reviewing and recalling" the day's experiences, which helps transfer information into your long-term memory. Sleep regulates your body clock, known as the "circadian rhythm," which is naturally attuned with the daily cycle of light and darkness, and is detected by your eyes. It is the reason why people suffer from jet lag after a long-haul flight, and it takes awhile for the body clock to readjust.

How much sleep?

The amount of sleep required varies from person to person. Some people can get by with as little as five hours a night, while others need nine. It is important to be aware of what your own "magic number" is and try to stick to that figure. Otherwise you risk inhibiting your productivity as well as your ability to remember and process information. A lack of sleep puts an enormous strain on the brain. Studies have shown that a sleep-deprived brain loses efficiency. An area usually active during a specific task needs to be propped up by other parts of the brain. It is like driving a vehicle with a flat tire—your performance is severely reduced. Sleep deprivation also increases stress hormone levels, which reduces nerve cell production (neurogenesis) in the adult brain.

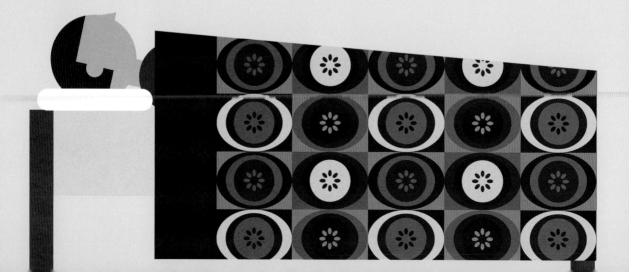

Stages of sleep

Sleep can be divided into four separate brain stages. There's the *theta* wave when we sometimes rouse with a sudden jerk. Then there's the *delta* wave activity, during which if awoken you'd be totally disorientated. While asleep you go back and forth through these two brainwave patterns in 90-minute cycles. It is then that you also enter REM sleep, where your eyelids show movement of a seemingly alert mind. And then, of course, there's the dream state which, according to Freud, acts as a safety valve for the overburdened brain.

Top tips for good sleep

• Establish regular times—get used to your body-clock even on weekends, when you are tempted to sleep in.

• Avoid caffeine, alcohol, and nicotine before bedtime—all of which disrupt natural sleep patterns.

• Finish eating at least three hours before regular bedtime.

• Exercise daily, although not too close to bedtime.

• Use relaxing bedtime rituals such as soaking in a hot tub, or scented candles; listen to soothing music an hour or more before you aim to fall asleep.

• Keep your bedroom a *bedroom*, not a study or a TV room.

• Try to keep out light and noise.

• Make sure your mattress and pillows are comfortable.

• Don't try to force sleep. If you can't fall asleep within 15–20 minutes of going to bed, do something distracting. Get out of bed and make a cup of caffeine-free tea or read a magazine.

Nap for a mini brain boost

If you feel drowsy in the early afternoon, perhaps after lunch, take a 20-minute nap. It might be impractical in many circumstances but it will do your brain more good than reaching for a cup of coffee. Daytime napping is healthy for the brain. You need it to refresh your brain cells and allow the different areas to recover. If your brain's tired, your performance will slow down. A nap is also a good de-stresser. Some researchers have even suggested that a six-minute nap can improve performances in memory and problem-solving tests.

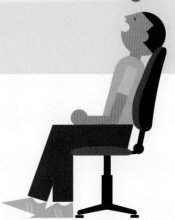

Brain food

There is an American proverb that says: "We need brain more than belly food," and it couldn't be more true. As we stated on page 12, a resting person's brain uses 20 percent of food energy even though it accounts for just two percent of the body's weight. Your brain needs fuel, especially foods packed with brain-boosting nutrients. Here are some top brain-training foods:

1. Salmon or other oily fish, which contain the omega-3 family of fatty acids, help maintain brain cells and build stronger and better connections between them.

2. Brightly colored fruit and vegetables, notably blueberries and spinach, are high in antioxidants that can also maintain healthy brain cells and improve brain-cell connectivity.

3. Avocado is one of the most easily digestible sources of high-quality protein and healthy fats. Avocado also contains antioxidants, fiber, and folate, among other nutrients.

4. Nuts contain protein, complex carbohydrates, and beneficial fats. They also provide a good dose of vitamin E, which promotes brain function. Almonds are the best nuts, followed by hazelnuts, cashews, pistachios, and walnuts.

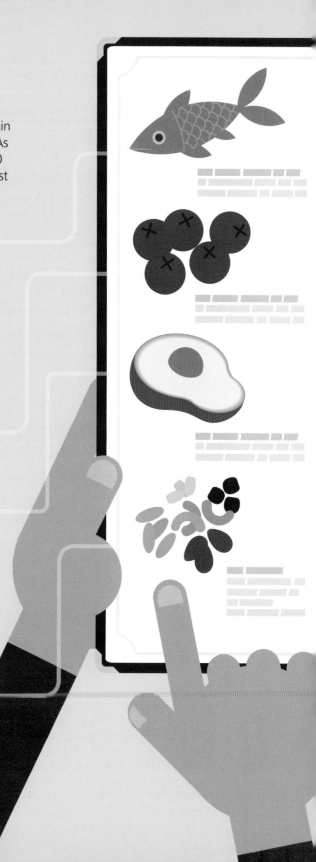

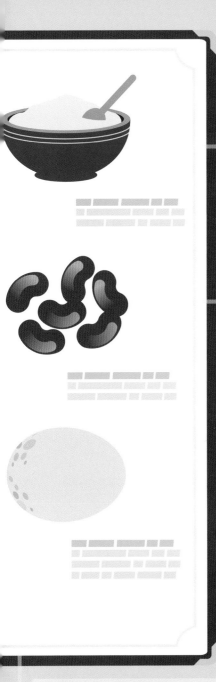

Alcohol

It's common knowledge nowadays that a daily glass of wine helps you de-stress, but did you know about the study that revealed that drinking alcohol can actually boost your brainpower?

The study, conducted by the Australian National University in Canberra, monitored 7,000 people in their early 20s, 40s, and 60s, and found that those who drank within safe limits (no more than two drinks per day for men and one drink per day for women) had better verbal skills, memory, and speed of thinking than those who either drank excessively or not at all. How might alcohol be boosting brainpower? Some experts believe that the cardiovascular benefits of alcohol might extend to the brain. However, the researchers were quick to point out that although the results were surprising, they do not necessarily prove for certain that alcohol benefits the brain, since the study did not consider all the potential reasons why the nondrinkers performed less well than the drinkers. Medical professionals do acknowledge the potential health benefits of alcohol, but emphasize that it should be regarded as a double-edged sword because the risk of abuse is high and the consequences of binge-drinking and alcoholism are well documented throughout the world.

5. Oats promote healthy blood flow to help your brain function better. They also contain fiber, protein, antioxidants, and some omega-3 acids.

6. Beans and legumes are loaded with fiber, vitamins, minerals, protein, and folic acid, and give your brain a slow, stable supply of glucose.

Dark chocolate

Dark chocolate is a beneficial brain food! It contains magnesium, which increases the supply of oxygen to the brain, and high levels of polyphenols, an antioxidant chemical that reduces blood pressure. Raw cocoa has the highest antioxidant value of all the natural foods in the world—twice the antioxidants of red wine, and up to three times the antioxidants found in green tea. It also appears to regulate levels of the feel-good chemical serotonin in the brain. Scientists followed up an examination of 10 patients who received 1.6 oz of dark chocolate daily for two months. Patients given the dark chocolate reported less Chronic Fatigue Syndrome (CFS) and claimed to feel the weariness return when they stopped taking it.

7. Eggs contain protein and fat and are another source of stable energy for your brain. The selenium in organic eggs has been shown to help improve mood. Choline, also found in eggs, is a protein, a building block of every cell, and has been linked to improved memory.

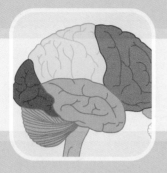
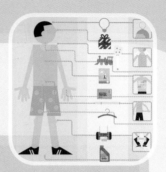
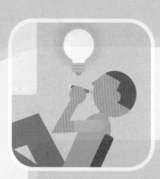
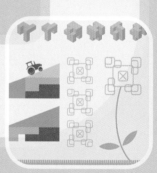
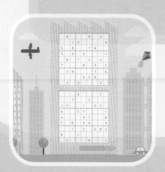
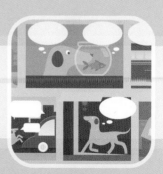

Chapter 8

Test your new brainpower

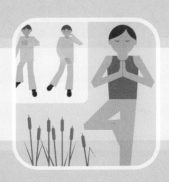 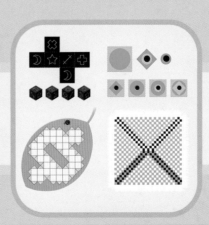

→ Final workout

You'll find an assortment of exercises throughout the next 10 pages that will test your memory, visual, creative, numerical, and verbal skills. You'll be given a score for each exercise you complete correctly. Add up the scores at the end to find out your new mental agility.

1. Number recall

Study this picture for 1 minute, paying close attention to the numbers on the soccer jerseys. Now cover up the image and answer the questions below:

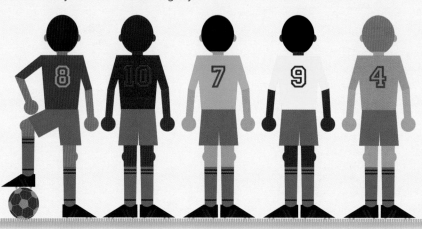

A: What total do you get when you add up the even-numbered jerseys?

B: What total do you get when you add up the odd-numbered jerseys?

C: What is the color of the jersey with the number 9 on it?

D: What number is printed on the blue jersey?

E: What total do you get when you add up the numbers on all the jerseys?

•1 point for each correct answer

2. The correct cube

If you folded the template into a cube, which of the 4 options underneath might you see?

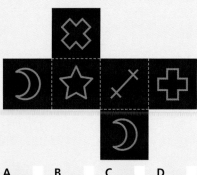

A   B   C   D

•1 point

3. Old mates

Mr. Smith is walking down the street when he bumps into an old classmate who he hasn't seen for 20 years, and who is pushing a carriage with a little girl inside.

"Oh, you have a daughter!" Smith says to his old pal. "Are you married then?"

"Yes," the schoolmate replies.

"To whom?"

"Someone you don't know," his friend replies.

"And what's the name of your daughter?" Smith asks.

"It's the same as her mother's."

"Then this little girl must be called Lucy!" Smith concludes.

"That's right!"

How did Mr. Smith guess the little girl's name?

•2 points

4. Number grid

This is a basic test of mental arithmetic. Fill in the number grid with the correct functions to get the answers for each row and column. Time yourself

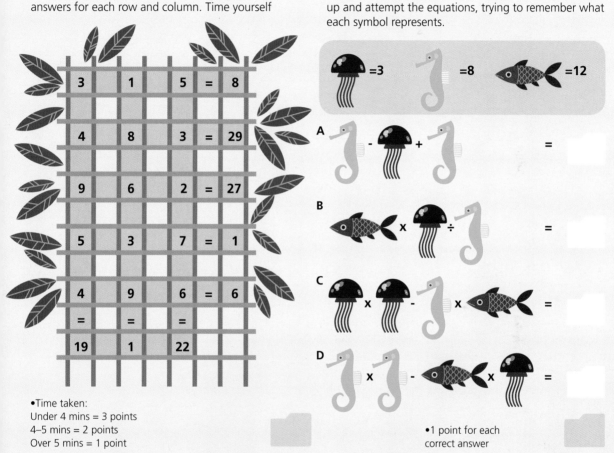

3		1		5	=	8
4		8		3	=	29
9		6		2	=	27
5		3		7	=	1
4		9		6	=	6
=		=		=		
19		1		22		

•Time taken:
Under 4 mins = 3 points
4–5 mins = 2 points
Over 5 mins = 1 point

6. Memory math

The numbers have been replaced by the symbols below. Study the symbols for 30 seconds, and then cover them up and attempt the equations, trying to remember what each symbol represents.

(jellyfish) =3   (seahorse) =8   (fish) =12

A.   (seahorse) − (jellyfish) + (seahorse)   =

B.   (fish) × (jellyfish) ÷ (seahorse)   =

C.   (jellyfish) × (jellyfish) − (seahorse) × (fish)   =

D.   (seahorse) × (seahorse) − (fish) × (jellyfish)   =

•1 point for each correct answer

5. Colored words

Read out loud the color the word is printed in. Try to do it in the quickest time possible.

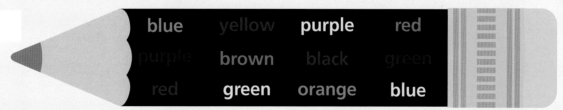

blue   yellow   **purple**   red
purple   **brown**   black   green
red   **green**   orange   **blue**

•Time taken:
Under 12 secs = 3 points
13–16 secs = 2 points
Over 17 secs = 1 point

Solutions on p.184 >>>

7. Squaring up: part two

If you remove 2 shapes from this assortment, you can piece the rest together to form a square. Identify the 2 shapes you will need to remove.

A

B   C   D

E   F

•2 points

8. Matchstick mayhem

Make the animal look in the opposite direction by moving 2 matchsticks and its eye, making sure its tail is still pointing up.

•2 points

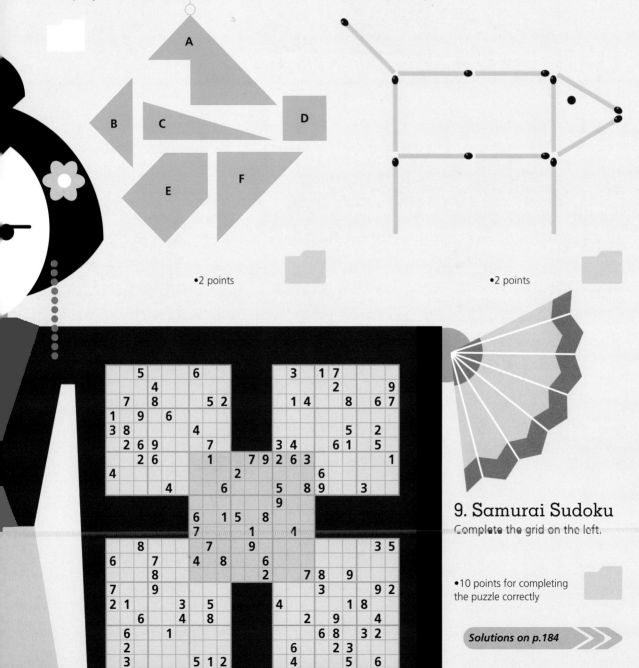

9. Samurai Sudoku

Complete the grid on the left.

•10 points for completing the puzzle correctly

Solutions on p.184 »

10. The word ladder

Use word association to move up the ladder to the final word.

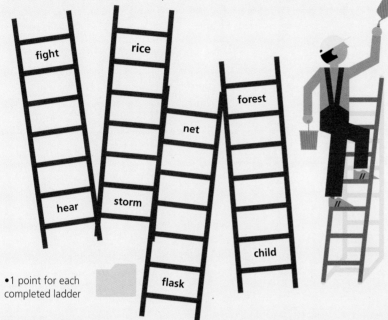

fight

rice

forest

net

storm

hear

child

flask

• 1 point for each completed ladder

11. Hungry lion

Imagine you have been captured and suspended from a tree. The rope is anchored to the ground and a candle is slowly burning through the rope. There is a hungry lion waiting for you to drop so that he can eat you. You don't have the strength to flip up and untie the rope, reach up to the branch, or even swing over to the trunk. Help will be on its way in about an hour. What can you do to prevent yourself being eaten by the lion?

• 2 points

12. Shooting arrows

Mary, Thomas, and Carla took part in an archery contest. Mary shot the pink arrows, Thomas shot the green arrows, and Carla shot the blue arrows. You can see how each of them fared in the diagram.

A: How many points did Thomas score?

B: What is Mary and Carla's combined total?

C: During the third round Mary hit a 9-point shot. However, it later transpired that her foot crossed the line and that effort was disqualified. How many points did she score after the amendment?

D: Which player won (after amendment)?

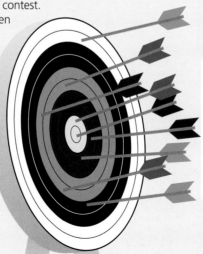

Working from the center outward, the colors and points are:

Gold inner	10
Gold outer	9
Red inner	8
Red outer	7
Blue inner	6
Blue outer	5
Black inner	4
Black outer	3
White inner	2
White outer	1

Mary

Thomas

Carla

• 1 point for each correct answer

13. Scrambled sentences

Unscramble the words in each of the following to make a proper sentence:

A: and memory Daily concentration exercises skills boost can

B: refrigerator brain light as about a energy much Your uses as

C: ticklish tickle No how be you might you yourself can't matter

D: instrument spatial Learning play improves to musical reasoning a

E: health and a brain good maintains exercise Physical diet

F: vivid events intense memories Emotionally produce

G: awareness feeling others of what depend are skills Social the on

•1 point for each correct answer

14. Recall the flags

Study these flags for 1 minute, then cover them up and write the name of the country in the grid provided.

Belgium   India   USA   China   UK   Netherlands   Germany   France

•1 point for each correct answer

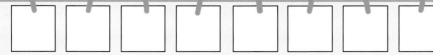

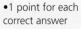

15. Stacking mosaic tiles

If you placed these shapes on top of each other, starting with the largest at the bottom, which image would you see?

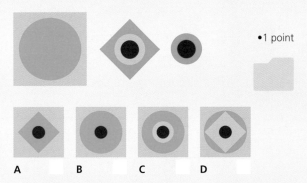

A   B   C   D

• 1 point

16 Quick-fire riddles

A: How many times can you subtract the number 5 from 25?

B: What gets whiter the dirtier it gets?

C: What do you possess but other people use it more than you do?

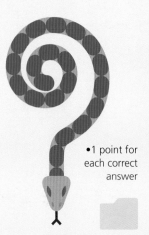

• 1 point for each correct answer

17. Krazy Kakuro

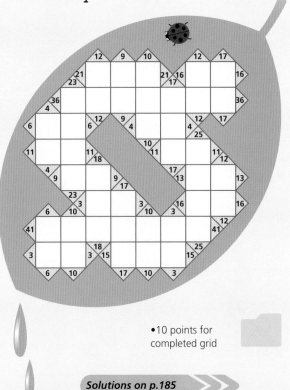

• 10 points for completed grid

Solutions on p.185

• 1 point for each correct answer

18. Spot the errors

Find the word that is spelled incorrectly in each sentence and write the correct spelling in the answer box.

A: The baby waeled throughout the church service.

B: He was an accessery to the crime.

C: They accomdated us really well during our vacation.

D: Phillip was definitely unaccusstomed to public speaking.

E: The weather looks very changgable.

F: The teacher was very dissappointed.

G: The television was cheap but came without a guarantie.

19. A love of animals

At a board meeting the 12 directors of a popular zoo are talking about their favorite animals. Study the diagram for 1 minute and then cover it up and answer the following questions:

A: What is Mr. Mukherjee's favorite animal?

B: Which director's favorite animal is the giraffe?

C: Which 2 animals are mentioned that belong to the cat family?

D: Who is sitting to the left of the person whose favorite animal is a panda?

E: What is Mr. Alves' favorite animal?

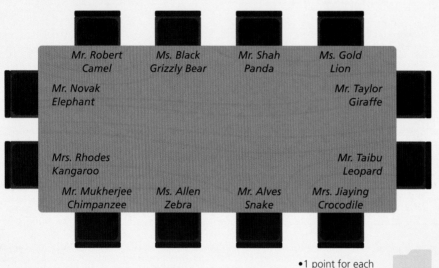

Mr. Robert Camel	Ms. Black Grizzly Bear	Mr. Shah Panda	Ms. Gold Lion
Mr. Novak Elephant			Mr. Taylor Giraffe
Mrs. Rhodes Kangaroo			Mr. Taibu Leopard
Mr. Mukherjee Chimpanzee	Ms. Allen Zebra	Mr. Alves Snake	Mrs. Jiaying Crocodile

•1 point for each correct answer

20. Complete the cube

Which 2 shapes will pair up to create the top shape?

•1 point

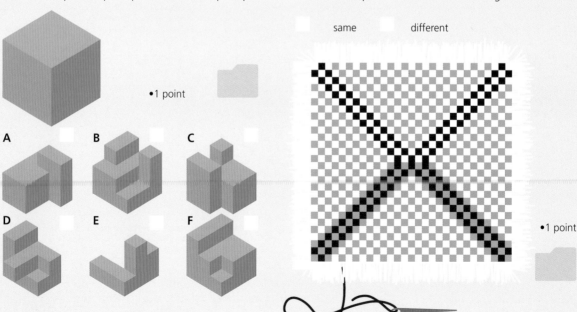

A   B   C

D   E   F

21. Colored squares

Are the red squares the same color throughout the "X"?

same   different

•1 point

22. Shopping task

You're in a clothes shop buying items of clothing to go on vacation. You bought 11 items, paid $150 and got $3.10 change. How many of each item did you buy?

Tops:

Skirts:

Socks:

Belts: •3 points

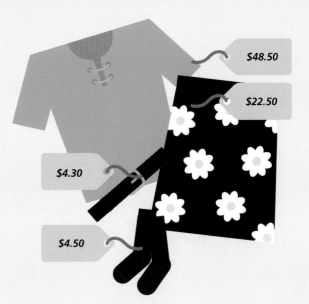

$48.50

$22.50

$4.30

$4.50

23. Locate the loot

In jail, Tony's cellmate told him that he had buried the loot from a heist in a secret location, and showed him a map he'd drawn to keep a note of the location. Later on, Tony stole the map from under his cellmate's pillow and had only 1 minute to memorize the route before his cellmate returned. Assuming that you are Tony, study the footsteps on the map below for 1 minute and then cover it up and draw it on the empty grid.

•1 point for the correct route

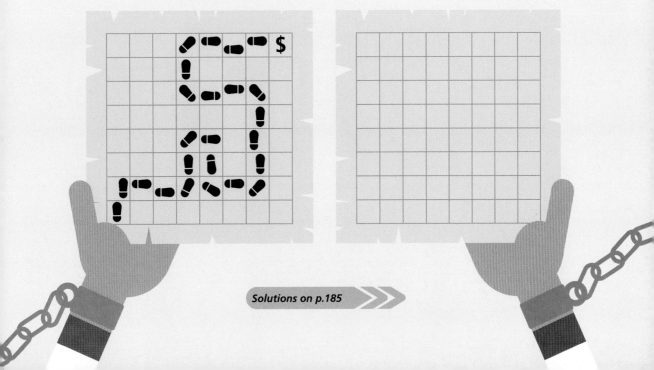

Solutions on p.185

24. Build the bird

All of these pieces can be put together to form the picture of the bird below. Draw the individual pieces in the grid provided.

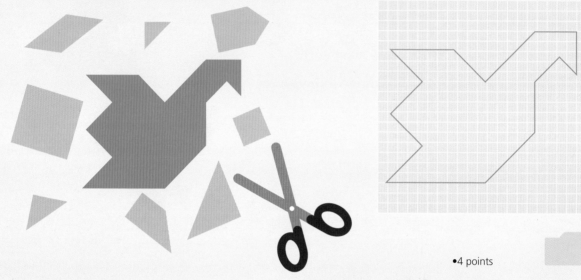

•4 points

25. Suitor challenge

Four suitors approached a hotel magnate asking for his daughter's hand in marriage. The hotelier thought of a way to test his suitors. The suitor to pass the test would receive his daughter's hand in marriage.

The daughter was put in the center of a large banquet room. The four suitors were put in each corner of the room on top of a podium. The first one to touch the daughter's hand would be the winner and become his son-in-law.

The rules of the test were that the suitors could not walk over the carpet, cross the plane of the carpet, or hang from anything; nor could they use anything but their body and wits (no magic or telepathy, nor any items such as ladders, block and tackles, and so on).

One suitor figured out a way and married the hotelier's daughter. What did he do?

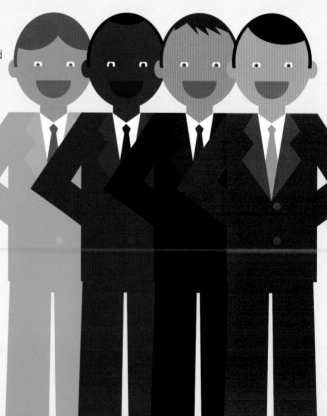

•2 points

26. Fitting jigsaw puzzle pieces

What can you see when you arrange these jigsaw puzzle pieces correctly?

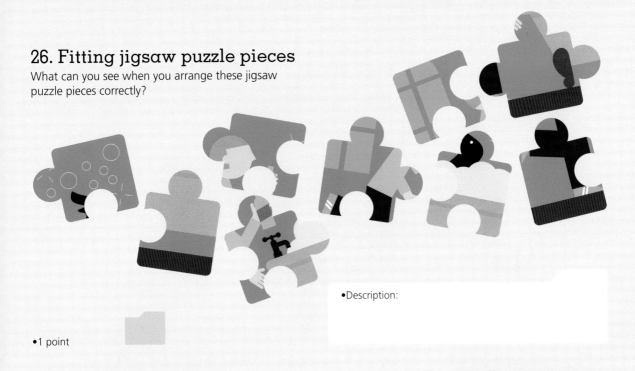

•Description:

•1 point

27. The shortest route

Find the shortest path possible through the grid. We've given you a head start. Can you finish it?

Solutions on p.185

finish

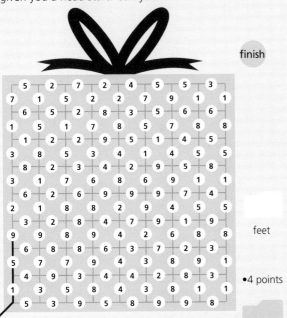

feet

•4 points

start

How did you do?

It's time to add up your points. Turn to pages 184–185 for the answers and figure out your score. There is a total of 100 points up for grabs.

YOUR SCORE: /100

How did you do in this final workout? How does your new score compare to the points you earned in the first chapter? Did you find that the puzzles were easier with all the tips, strategies, and techniques at your disposal? We'd like to stress that your brain workout shouldn't stop here. Regular brain training will ensure that you develop clearer and quicker thinking power, improved memory, increased focus, and an overall sense of well-being.

Solutions

1: Brain potential

2. Number sequences
A: 768 (x 4 each time)
B: 13 (add the preceding two numbers in the sequence)
C: 37 (a sub-sequence of ascending odd numbers drives this sequence, which is added each time)
2   5   10   17   26   37
    3   5   7   9   11
D: 253 (x 2 + 3 each time)

3. Building fences
B

4. Goat, cabbage, and wolf
The farmer ferries the goat over first. He returns and takes the cabbage. He deposits the cabbage on the other side and takes the goat back. He then leaves the goat and picks up the wolf. He ferries the wolf to the other side. Finally, he returns to pick up the goat again.

5. Mental arithmetic
A: 9   **F:** 32   **K:** 9
B: 17   **G:** 5   **L:** 9
C: 20   **H:** 72   **M:** 40
D: 12   **I:** 42   **N:** 12
E: 49   **J:** 16   **O:** 24

6. A perfect circle?
The inner circle is perfect. Sometimes it's difficult to see the wood for the trees, and the "information" around the object you are interested in can distort your view. Try covering the lines with a card, and you will see that the circle is perfect.

8. Dog and bone

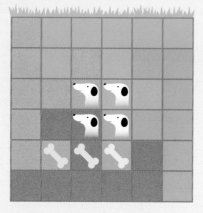

9. Light switches
Turn the left switch on for 10 minutes then turn it off again. Turn the middle switch on and go upstairs. The light turned on matches the middle switch. Carefully touch the other two bulbs. The one that's hot matches the left switch, the cool one matches the right.

11. Spot the differences

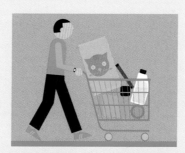

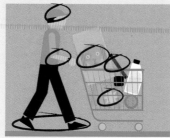

12. Numerical jigsaw

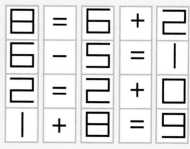

13. Visual logic test
C: The other shapes have 4 straight lines
C: The other shapes consist of a square, a circle and a triangle
D: This has 6 arrowhead shapes, while the others have only 5

14. Manhole covers
1. A square manhole cover can be turned and dropped down the diagonal of the manhole. This will not happen with a round manhole cover. So, for safety and practicality, all manhole covers should be round.
2. Another answer is that a round manhole cover can be rolled around to save having to lift it.

15. Moving by degrees
1 degree

16. Motorcycle parts
C

17. Straight lines
Both horizontal lines are straight. Similar to exercise 6, your view is distorted by the circle of lines receding to the vanishing point. Your eyes focus on the vanishing point, and this causes the two straight lines to appear warped.

19. Magic square

6	7	2
1	5	9
8	3	4

20. Color mazes
A:

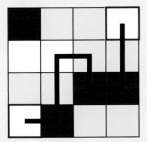

B:

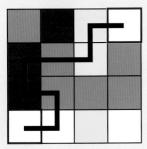

C:

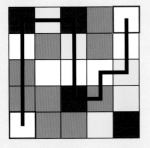

21. A perfectly boiled egg
Turn both timers upside down and put the egg into the boiling water. After 7 minutes, turn the 7-minute timer. Then when 11 minutes have passed, turn the 7-minute timer again. Then it will take another 4 minutes until the 7-minute timer stops. At that time, exactly 15 minutes have passed.

22. Spot the odd picture
A: Feet (the rest are parts of the face)
B: Bread slice (the rest are whole)
C: Plank of wood (the rest can be melted)
D: Gold (the rest are precious stones)
E: Pen (the rest convey information)

23. Odd word out
A: Fish (the rest are land animals)
B: Stream (the rest are still waters)
C: Stool (the rest are raw materials)
D: Lawn (the rest are naturally occurring landscapes)
E: Corfu (the rest are names for the country of Cyprus in French, English and German

2: Memory

2. Attention to detail
A: The painting of the Mona Lisa has no eyebrows
B: The right hand rests on the left

4. Spot the changes

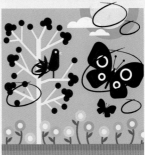

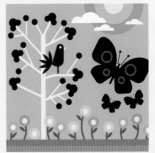

11. Where was that?
B

13. Sewing patterns
Most people should be able to remember more strokes in the second grid, simply because the brain identifies the representation of sea creatures and can, therefore, form a memory of them more easily.

14. Memory math
A: 8
B: 7
C: 56

15. Olympic colors
A: Blue
D: Green
E: Red

3: Visual reasoning and spatial awareness

1. Overlapped objects
A: Apple; wrench; stapler
B: Guitar; bicycle; car
C: Calculator; saw; yacht
D: Fish; pen; toothbrush

2. Guess the picture

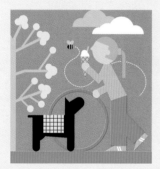

3. Triangle test
24

4. Spot the flipper
A: 2   **C:** 3
B: 3   **D:** 1

5. Cake for eight
All you need is 2 vertical and 1 horizontal cut

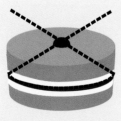

6. Reversed digits

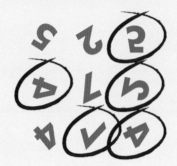

7. Quick-speed accounting
A: 33
B: 23 "3"s and 36 "7"s

8. Largest circle
A, B, and C, would have the same diameter.

9. Straight or crooked?
Straight

10. Phony image
D and F

11. Largest parcel?
They all have the same surface area.

12. Sharp fox
28 triangles

13. Counting stars
A: 5
B: 4
C: 3

14. Solitary snowflake

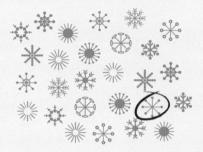

15. Find the treasure
D

16. Origami enigma
C

17. Shape shifting
C

18. Stacking mosaic tiles
A

19. Squaring up
C

20. The correct cube
C

21. False pattern
C

22. Perfect fit
B

23. On a roll
D

24. The vanishing area
Martin Gardner first described the vanishing area paradox in 1961. The paradox concerns a triangle constructed with 4 colored pieces. When the pieces are rearranged to form a second triangle, a tiny empty area appears.

   The answer to this problem is fairly simple. The 2 "triangles" are actually optical illusions, because the orange triangle and the green one are not in equal proportions. The green one is 8 x 3 squares, and the orange one is 5 x 2 squares. Therefore, in the 2 complex "triangles" the hypotenuse is not a straight line. In the first example it bends downward slightly, and in the second one it bends upward slightly. The difference between these two lines is the "extra" square in the lower drawing.

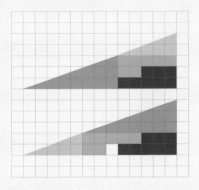

25. Spinning blossom
C

4: Think creatively

5. Horsing around
1. Only 3 of the 4 horses are his, so he only needs to lasso 3 to make sure that none of *his* horses remain untethered.
2. One of his horses is already tethered, so he only needs to throw the lasso over the 3 other horses.
3. The white horse is an inanimate carousel figure and therefore cannot escape. If you are prepared to open your mind, you'll find that there are other possibilities too.

6. Doubling the window size
1. Open the window.
2. Providing it's a double pane window, if you were to separate the panes, the window would become twice as large.
3. Put a giant magnifying glass in front of it.
4. Place a giant mirror at an angle beside it.

7. Enough fish
There was the father, his son, and his son's son. This equals 2 fathers and 2 sons!

8. Drinking glasses
You can solve the problem by moving a single glass. Simply pick up the middle one of the full glasses, pour the water into the middle one of the empty glasses, and return the glass to its original position.

9. The elder twin
At the time she went into labor, the mother of the twins was traveling by boat. The older twin, Terry, was born first, in the early hours on March 1st. The boat then crossed the International Date Line (or any time zone line) and Kerry, the younger twin, was born on February the 28th. In a leap year the younger twin celebrates her birthday two days before her older brother.

10. The swimmer in the forest
During a forest fire a fire-fighting plane had scooped up some water from the lake to drop on the fire. The plane had accidentally picked up the swimmer as well.

11. Crossing the bridge
One solution:

The singer and the guitarist cross = 2 mins (total = 2)
The singer goes back = 1 min (total = 3)
The drummer and the keyboardist cross = 10 mins (total = 13)
The guitarist goes back = 2 mins (total = 15)
The singer and the guitarist cross = 2 mins (total = 17)
An alternative solution is to swap the singer with the guitarist.

12. The third square

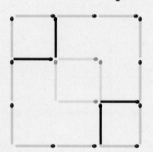

13. Three for two

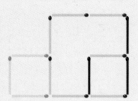

14. Remove a square

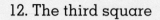

15. Swimming fish

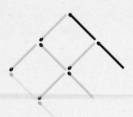

16. Try for five

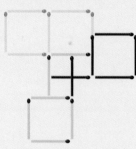

17. Even out

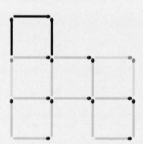

18. All the threes

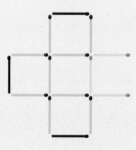

19. Total wipeout

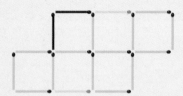

20. Equal divide

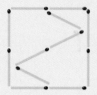

21. Find the extra triangle

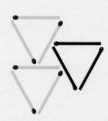

22. Break the wheel

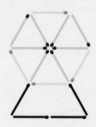

23. More for less

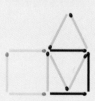

24. Ice in the glass

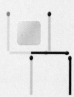

25. Doubling up

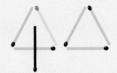

26. The elusive square

27. Two's company

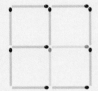

28. Polar explorer
1. Scott Amundsen Peary drove his car for 1 mile in reverse.
2. If the road is icy enough, he could spin his wheels, measure the distance on the odometer, and wind up in the same place he started.
3. The road curves around.

29. A son's gratitude
The son, in his late teens, was spoiled and idle. The father believed that evicting him and forcing him to find his own way through life would benefit him, however unpleasant it would be at first, and so threw him out. When the son found a job and worked his way up the career ladder, he understood how his father's action had made his life constructive and successful. Therefore, he returned to thank his father.

30. Deadly shell
Aeschylus died when the tortoise was dropped on him from a height by an eagle that might have mistaken Aeschylus' bald head for a rock on which to break the tortoise's shell.

31. Foiled robbery
Panic stricken, the bank robber dashed to the revolving door and tried to barge in the direction the door would not turn. The force of his own push knocked him to the ground, the weapon fell out of his hand, and a brave customer grabbed the gun.

32. Futile car chase
The getaway vehicle was a double-decker bus that went under a low bridge. The top deck of the bus was ripped off and fell over the pursuing police car.

33. Clever dunce
William's name was William Abbot and the results were given in alphabetical order.

34. The fatal flash
The man is a lion-tamer, posing for a photo with his lion. The lion reacts badly to the flash of the camera, and the man can't see properly, so he gets mauled.

35. Lax borders
He is a mailman who delivers packages to the different foreign embassies in the United States. The land of an embassy belongs to the country of the embassy, not to the United States.

36. Strange detour
The elevator only runs to the 7th floor. The riddle did not state that he takes the elevator from the 10th floor in the morning, just that he takes it to the first floor. He walks down to the 7th floor each morning to take the elevator to the first floor also.

37. Bottled money
Push the cork *into* the bottle, and shake out the coin.

38. Separated at birth?
They were two of a set of triplets (or quadruplets, and so on).

39. Push that car
The man pushing the car was a player in a Monopoly game and his gamepiece was a car.

40. Newspaper divider
Tom's mother slid the newspaper under a closed door, and made each sibling stand on either side of it.

41. Nail on the tree
The nail would remain at the same height since trees grow at their tops.

42. The café wall
The "Café Wall" illusion was first reported by Richard L. Gregory and Priscilla Heard in 1979, after they noticed it in the pattern of tiles on a café wall in Bristol. The illusion gives the impression that the tiles are wedge-shaped because the grout lines appear to slope alternately upward and downward. However, if you were to align the tiles, you will see that the lines are actually parallel, and all the tiles are perfectly square and of the same size.

43. Big-headed flower
This is called the Ebbinghaus illusion (also known as the "Titchener illusion")—it's an optical illusion of relative size perception. The 2 circles of identical size are placed near each other; larger circles surround one while smaller circles surround the other. The first central circle then appears smaller than the second central circle. The Ebbinghaus illusion provides a valuable way to investigate how the eye and brain process visual information.

44. Confused creature

This illusion offers up an ambiguous illustration in which the brain switches between seeing a rabbit and a duck. The duck-rabbit was originally noted by American psychologist Joseph Jastrow in 1899. Jastrow used the drawing to point out that perception is not just a product of the stimulus, but also of mental activity.

45. Dotty or what?

This is called the Hermann grid illusion. It is characterized by "ghostlike" gray blobs perceived at the intersections of a white (or light-colored) grid on a black background. The gray blobs disappear when you look directly at an intersection.

46. Look into my tie ...

This is one of many versions of the rolling wave illusion. Because our eyes and minds have been hardwired by evolution to identify patterns and relationships to help recognize the world around us, they can be fooled by images that seemingly replicate those patterns and relationships. When you stare at this illusion, the brain is being fooled and is failing to re-create the physical world.

47. Poles apart

This is a version of the twisted cord illusion. The horizontal lines seen contain obvious sloping elements. This information takes precedence, which the eyes transfer to the brain, so despite the poles being parallel to each other, the brain only recognizes the sloping elements and deduces that the poles must be slanted.

5: Numerical reasoning

Quick-fire arithmetic test

1. c
2. a
3. a
4. b
5. a
6. a
7. b
8. a
9. b
10. c
11. b
12. a
13. b
14. b
15. c
16. a
17. c
18. b
19. c
20. b
21. c
22. b
23. c
24. a
25. c
26. b
27. a
28. a
29. b
30. a
31. c
32. b
33. a
34. c
35. c

1. Under the bridge
54 ft

2. Casting shadows
A: 90 ft
B: 202½ ft

3. Wedding fit
A: January
B: Tara
C: Tara

4. Chance amour
10 seconds
The man would have progressed 90 ft and the woman, 30 ft.

5. Keen student
A: 2 miles
B: 3 miles
C: 24 mph

6. Carrying cupcakes

Small tray	24 cakes
Medium tray	40 cakes
Large tray	48 cakes

7. Land up for grabs
A: 5,184 ft^2
B: 2,592 ft^2
C: 3,456 ft^2
D: $3,840
E: $11,520

8. Bathroom makeover
A: ⅐
B: 7 packs
C: $16.80

9. Computer sales
A: May
B: 27 percent
C: 1,050 units

10. The shortest route
39 yards

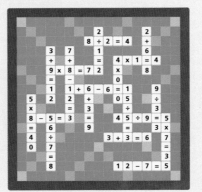

11. The broken calculator

2 = 0.5 x 4	9 = 4 + 5
3 = 0.5 x 5 + 0.5	10 = 5 x 2
4 = 2 x 2	11 = 2 + 4 + 5
5 = 2.5 x 2	12 = 3 x 4
6 = 2 x 3	13 = 5 x 2 + 3
7 = 4 + 3	14 = 5 x 2 + 4
8 = 4 x 2	15 = 5 x 3

12. Unfold the folds
32 x 28 in
Each stage of unfolding:
1 = 8 x 7
2 = 8 x 14
3 = 16 x 14
4 = 16 x 28
5 = 32 x 28

13. Triangle ratio
You don't need to do any complicated mathematics. If you rotate the inner triangle by 180 degrees it should become obvious quickly that the ratio is 1:4.

14. Cross math

Intermediate Sudoku
Grid C

6	4	3	5	2	8	1	9	7
9	7	1	6	3	4	2	5	8
5	2	8	9	7	1	4	6	3
3	1	9	2	5	6	8	7	4
4	8	5	7	1	3	6	2	9
7	6	2	4	8	9	3	1	5
2	3	4	1	9	5	7	8	6
8	5	7	3	6	2	9	4	1
1	9	6	8	4	7	5	3	2

Easy Sudoku
Grid A

7	8	4	5	2	6	1	3	9
2	3	9	1	7	8	5	4	6
6	1	5	3	4	9	7	8	2
3	4	7	8	1	2	6	9	5
5	6	8	4	9	7	3	2	1
1	9	2	6	3	5	4	7	8
9	5	3	2	6	4	8	1	7
8	2	1	7	5	3	9	6	4
4	7	6	9	8	1	2	5	3

Grid D

1	8	5	6	4	3	9	7	2
3	6	7	9	5	2	8	1	4
2	9	4	8	1	7	5	3	6
6	2	9	5	7	8	3	4	1
4	5	3	2	9	1	7	6	8
7	1	8	3	6	4	2	9	5
9	7	1	4	2	5	6	8	3
8	4	2	7	3	6	1	5	9
5	3	6	1	8	9	4	2	7

Grid B

1	6	2	3	7	4	5	8	9
8	3	4	5	2	9	7	1	6
7	5	9	1	6	8	3	2	4
4	9	1	8	3	7	2	6	5
3	7	6	4	5	2	8	9	1
2	8	5	9	1	6	4	3	7
6	2	8	7	9	5	1	4	3
5	4	3	6	8	1	9	7	2
9	1	7	2	4	3	6	5	8

Hard Sudoku
Grid E

2	8	7	5	3	1	6	4	9
5	1	4	6	9	2	7	3	8
6	9	3	4	8	7	5	2	1
7	5	1	2	4	9	8	6	3
4	3	8	7	6	5	1	9	2
9	6	2	8	1	3	4	5	7
1	2	5	3	7	4	9	8	6
3	7	6	9	5	8	2	1	4
8	4	9	1	2	6	3	7	5

Samurai Sudoku

Grid A

```
9 2 5 7 6 1 8 4 3     1 8 7 5 3 4 9 6 2
8 7 3 4 5 9 2 1 6     3 4 6 2 9 7 1 8 5
6 4 1 3 2 8 9 5 7     9 2 5 8 1 6 4 7 3
5 8 2 9 3 6 4 7 1     8 9 1 6 4 5 3 2 7
7 6 4 8 1 2 5 3 9     7 5 4 3 8 2 6 1 9
1 3 9 5 7 4 6 2 8     6 3 2 1 7 9 8 5 4
4 1 7 6 9 5 3 8 2  5 1 3  4 6 9 7 2 1 5 3 8
2 9 8 1 4 3 7 6 5  9 4 7  2 1 8 4 5 3 7 9 6
3 5 6 2 8 7 1 9 4  8 2 6  5 7 3 9 6 8 2 4 1
                   4 1 9 6 3 5 8 2 7
                   8 2 6 1 7 4 9 3 5
                   5 7 3 2 8 9 1 4 6
1 9 3 5 7 2 6 4 8  7 9 2  3 5 1 7 9 2 8 4 6
4 2 5 6 1 8 9 3 7  4 5 1  6 8 2 3 4 1 5 9 7
6 8 7 3 4 9 2 5 1  3 6 8  7 9 4 6 8 5 3 2 1
8 5 6 1 3 4 7 9 2            4 2 8 5 3 6 1 7 9
9 7 4 8 2 5 1 6 3            9 7 6 8 1 4 2 3 5
2 3 1 9 6 7 5 8 4            1 3 5 2 7 9 6 8 4
7 6 2 4 9 3 8 1 5            2 1 7 9 6 8 4 5 3
3 1 8 2 5 6 4 7 9            8 4 3 1 5 7 9 6 2
5 4 9 7 8 1 3 2 6            5 6 9 4 2 3 7 1 8
```

Grid B

```
8 7 4 3 2 6 9 1 5     4 8 3 5 7 6 2 9 1
2 1 9 5 4 7 3 8 6     1 7 6 4 9 2 5 3 8
3 6 5 1 9 8 7 4 2     9 2 5 8 1 3 7 4 6
1 9 8 6 3 2 4 5 7     6 1 9 2 5 4 8 7 3
5 4 2 8 7 1 6 9 3     7 4 8 9 3 1 6 5 2
7 3 6 9 5 4 1 2 8     3 5 2 7 6 8 4 1 9
4 2 1 7 8 3 5 6 9  4 7 2  8 3 1 6 4 7 9 2 5
6 5 7 2 1 9 8 3 4  1 6 5  2 9 7 1 8 5 3 6 4
9 8 3 4 6 5 2 7 1  3 8 9  5 6 4 3 2 9 1 8 7
                   6 2 5 8 4 7 9 1 3
                   7 1 8 9 3 6 4 5 2
                   9 4 3 5 2 1 7 8 6
5 6 9 3 4 7 1 8 2  7 9 3  6 4 5 2 8 9 1 3 7
4 1 8 2 5 6 3 9 7  6 5 4  1 2 8 5 3 7 6 9 4
3 7 2 9 8 1 4 5 6  2 1 8  3 7 9 4 6 1 2 5 8
7 8 5 6 1 4 2 3 9            5 3 2 7 9 6 8 4 1
1 2 6 7 3   8 4 5            7 1 6 8 4 3 5 2 9
9 4 3 8 2 5 7 6 1            8 9 4 1 5 2 7 9 3
2 9 4 5 7 3 6 1 8            2 6 3 9 7 8 4 1 5
6 3 7 1 9 8 5 2 4            4 8 1 3 2 5 9 7 6
8 5 1 4 6 2 9 7 3            9 5 7 6 1 4 3 8 2
```

Kakuro games

Grid A

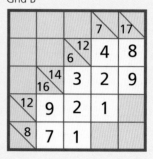

- Clues: 16, 7
- 13 : 9 4   (6)
- 11 : 7 1 3   (16)
- 12 : 2 1 9
- 9 : 2 7

Grid B

- Clues: 7, 17
- 12, (6) : 4 8
- 14, 16 : 3 2 9
- 12 : 9 2 1
- 8 : 7 1

Grid C

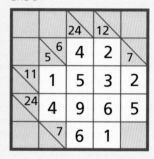

- Clues: 15, 26, 15
- 17 : 6 8 3
- 21 : 9 7 5   (12)
- 23 : 9 6 8
- 7 : 2 1 4

Grid D

- Clues: 24, 12
- 5, (6) : 4 2   (7)
- 11 : 1 5 3 2
- 24 : 4 9 6 5
- 7 : 6 1

Grid E

- Clues: 23, 7
- 8 : 6 2   (7)(23)
- 19 : 8 1 4 6
- 23 : 9 4 2 8
- 10 : 1 9

Grid F

- Clues: 24, 6
- (11) : 9 2
- 7, 24
- 20 : 1 9 7 3
- 18 : 2 7 8 1
- 12 : 4 8

15. Lottery numbers

This is known as the neglect of probability bias. It is a type of cognitive bias when one has a tendency to completely disregard probability when making a decision under uncertainty. Mathematically speaking, the numbers 1, 2, 3 ,4, 5, 6 are just as likely to come up as any other combination of numbers. Yet, people apply emotion and tend to pick numbers they feel they have a special connection with, such as birthdays, anniversary dates and "lucky" numbers.

16. Beer money

In psychology, this is called effort heuristic. It is a bias in which the value given to an object is based on the amount of perceived effort that went into producing the object. In our example, the $50 found in the street is considered less valuable because no effort has been made to earn the money, although that money has exactly the same monetary value as $50 earned by working at the coal mine, for example.

17. Bidding war

This is a case that demonstrates the concept of scarcity heuristics. In human psychology, this is a mental heuristic in which the mind values something based on how easily it may lose it, especially to competitors. Auctions operate on this concept. The auctioneer assigns a relatively low value to an object and hopes that several bidders will be interested enough to begin outbidding each other, thereby raising the value of the object.

18. Expensive tastes

Psychologists have identified a penchant for people to perceive more expensive goods as being better than inexpensive ones (providing they are of similar quality and style). They found this even holds true when prices and brands are switched—putting the high price on the normally relatively inexpensive brand is enough to lead people to perceive it as being better than the other product that is normally more expensive.

19. Bad luck?

You both have exactly the same chance, irrespective of how many times red has already come up.

20. Heads or tails?

The odds of it remain unchanged, at 50-50.

The misconception is that, given a set of possible alternative outcomes, namely, heads or tails, the distribution of said outcomes will tend to be even, or "average out," with repetition over time.

Belief in The Law of Averages is particularly prevalent in games of chance, in all of which cases it is entirely false, owing to the fact that the outcome of previous games has no bearing on the next game.

For instance, if "heads" lands for the first 10 tosses, intuition will suggest that, because tails has not come up in the last 10 tosses of the coin, it must therefore have a high probability of coming up next. This is false. In reality, it has the same probability as at any other throw. There is no causal link between previous throws and the next. History does not come into it.

21. Number sequences

A: 13112221—*Each line describes the previous sequence.*
1

11—one number one
21—two number ones
1211—one number two and one number one
111221—one number one, one number two, two number ones
312211—one number three, three number ones, two number twos, one number one.
B: 30—*The sequence follows the number of days in the months of the year, Jan = 31, Feb = 28, March = 31, and so on.*
C: 5—*The sequence follows the digits of Pi.*
D: 1—*This is an exception because it does follow mathematical logic.*

Do you see what comes next? First we took SIX to a power of ONE, then FIVE to the power of TWO, then FOUR to the power of THREE, and so on. Thus, the next number in the sequence equates to: 1x1x1x1x1x1 = 1

22. Chasing cars

If you have written down a whole page full of mathematical formulas, then you have probably been thinking in the wrong direction for this puzzle. The 2 cars will meet each other after 1 hour, hence the bird has been flying for 1 hour. The bird has flown 80 miles when the cars meet.

23. The famous 3 doors conundrum

If you don't change your mind, you have a 1 in 3 chance of winning the car. If you do change your mind, you have a 2 in 3 chance of winning. Many people find this answer very hard to believe, but it's true. For more explanation, see this website: www.jimloy.com/puzz/monty.htm

24. Weighing marbles

Number the bags from 1 to 10.
Take 1 marble from bag 1,
Take 2 marbles from bag 2,
Take 3 marbles from bag 3, ...
Take 9 marbles from bag 9 and
Take 10 marbles from bag 10.

Now put them on the scale. There are 10 possible measurements. If all marbles weighed 1 ounce, the total would be 55 oz. But one or more marbles weigh 0.9 oz. So if you took one 0.9 oz marble, the total would be 54.9 oz, if you took two 0.9 oz marbles, 54.8 oz, and so on.

You know the total weight, so you know the number of 0.9 oz marbles you took. That is, if the total was 54.9 oz, you took one 0.9 oz marble. If the total was 54.8 oz, you took two 0.9 oz marbles. And so on. Now that you know how many 0.9 oz marbles you took, you know which bag they're in because you took 1 marble from bag 1, 2 marbles from bag 2, and so on.

So if the weight is:
54.9 oz— the bag with the 0.9 oz marbles is bag 1.
54.8 oz—the bag with the 0.9 oz marbles is bag 2.
54.1 oz— the bag with the 0.9 oz marbles is bag 9.
54. oz—the bag with the 0.9 oz marbles is bag 10.

25. The condemned prisoner conundrum

White. If you had a black disk, the other 2 prisoners would be able to see 1 black and 1 white. They would know neither of theirs was black, because otherwise someone would have been able to see 2 blacks. Since no one has yet said a word, yours must be white. (Naturally, they can use the same reasoning; the trick is to be quickest.)

26. Break up time

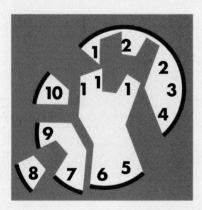

6: Verbal reasoning

1. Dictionary corner

1: A
2: B
3: A
4: B
5: A
6: C

2. Like for like

1: D	**8:** B
2: B	**9:** B
3: B	**10:** C
4: C	**11:** D
5: A	**12:** B
6: B	**13:** C
7: C	

3. Find the opposite

1: B	**6:** B
2: A	**7:** B
3: B	**8:** C
4: C	**9:** D
5: A	**10:** D

6. Scrambled sentences

A: Margaret is a strict schoolteacher
B: Physical exercise improves blood circulation to the brain
C: Your brain consists of about 100 billion neurons
D: Sudoku is a good brain-training exercise
E: The average reading speed is 200–250 words a minute
F: You are what you read
G: By reading you experience life vicariously through the eyes of another
H: Interviewers use verbal reasoning tests to find out how well a candidate can assess verbal logic

7: The word ladder

There can be any number of answers. Here's an example of how you could climb each ladder:
A: *umbrella —rain—sun—fire—candles—cake*
B: *bicycle—sport—race—time—stopwatch—clock*
C: *glasses—book—paper—tree—nest—bird*
D: *chair—desk—pen—letter—photograph—camera*

8. Word-play analogies

A: *departure*
B: *foot*
C: *above*
D: *animal*
E: *cold*

9. Student lodgings

A:
1: David
2: George
3: Harriet and Fiona
4: Emma

B:
5: Andrew and Fiona
6: George
7: George
8: House 2 (blue)

C:
9: David
10: Emma
11: David
12: Bruce

10. Odd one out

A: *Train*
A train travels on tracks. The rest travel on roads.
B: *Stocking*
A stocking is worn over the foot and leg. The rest are worn on the head.
C: *Tiger*
A tiger has stripes. The rest have spots.
D: *Log*
A log is a portion of a tree. The rest are rocks.

E: Tomato
A tomato is classified as a fruit. The rest are vegetables.
F: *Clarion*
A clarion is a wind instrument. The rest have a keyboard.

11. Spot the errors

Only last night, I **argued** with my **friend** about the correct **spelling** of a word: I said the correct spelling was "**committed**" while my friend insisted that it's "**committed.**" **Actually** I am surprised that people can make so many spelling errors. Often when you **point** out people's **mistakes** they feel criticized. Of **course**, the last thing I want to do is offend anybody; I just think it is good for **one's** personal **development** to improve **their** spelling. I've also found that if you point out **people's** spelling errors some people just get **embarrassed**, or **become** really defensive. I am **really** happy to report that the **college** I go to is **implementing** measures to tackle bad spelling; they are **drawing** up classes to teach students **how** to

assess what they read correctly. I think **it's wrong** for any teacher to ignore a student's bad spelling, and not **prepare them adequately** to go **out** into the wider world. We should, however, **remember** that bad spelling and bad thinking are **completely separate** issues. Just because **you're** a bad speller doesn't make you **dumb**. All it means is that you need to work harder to improve your spelling. It will really make a big **difference** when you start sending **your** CV to employers as to **whether** or not you get an interview.

12. Fill in the blanks

A: *Fireman*
B: *Mesmerizing*
C: *Bombarding*
D: *Extend*
E: *Expand*
F: *Trouncing*
G: *Scientist*

13. Wordy riddles

A: *Voice*
B: *One*—you have taken *one* cup of sugar
C: He said: *"You'll sentence me to 6 years in prison."*
If it were true then the judge would have to make it false by sentencing him to 4 years. If it were false, then he would have to give him 6 years, which would make it true. Rather than contradict his own word the judge set the man free.
D: *Time*

14. Summer job

Statement A—True
Statement B— False
Statement C—Cannot say

15. The sounds in my life

1: C
2: B
3: B
4: A
5: C
6: B
7: C

16. Dog's day out

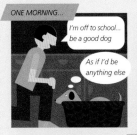
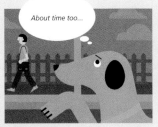
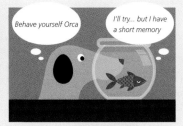
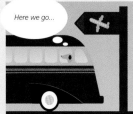
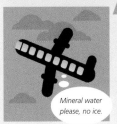
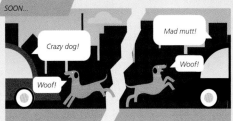
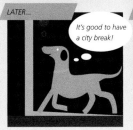
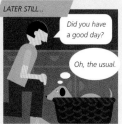

8: Test your new brainpower

1. Number recall
A: 22
B: 16
C: Yellow
D: 8
E: 38

2. The correct cube
D

3. Old friends
Mr. Smith's old classmate is called Lucy. In other words, he went to school with the mother.

4. Number grid

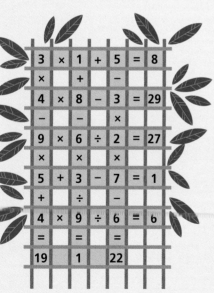

3	×	1	+	5	=	8
×		+		−		
4	×	8	−	3	=	29
−		−		×		
9	×	6	÷	2	=	27
×		×		×		
5	+	3	−	7	=	1
+		÷		−		
4	×	9	÷	6	=	6
=		=		=		
19		1		22		

6. Memory math
A: 13
B: 4.5
C: 12
D: 156

7. Squaring up: part two
C and D

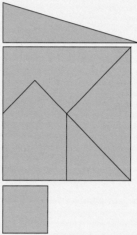

8. Matchstick mayhem

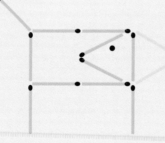

9. Samurai Sudoku

```
8 9 5 1 7 2 6 4 3        6 3 2 1 7 9 4 8 5
2 1 3 4 5 6 7 9 8        8 5 7 4 2 6 1 3 9
6 7 4 8 9 3 1 5 2        9 1 4 3 5 8 2 6 7
1 4 9 7 6 8 2 3 5        7 2 5 8 9 4 6 1 3
3 8 7 2 1 5 4 6 9        1 8 6 7 3 5 9 2 4
5 2 6 9 3 4 8 7 1        3 4 9 2 6 1 7 5 8
9 3 2 6 8 7 5 1 4 8 7 9 2 6 3 5 4 7 8 9 1
4 6 1 5 2 9 3 8 7 2 6 5 4 9 1 6 8 3 5 7 2
7 5 8 3 4 1 9 2 6 1 3 4 5 7 8 9 1 2 3 4 6
            8 4 3 6 2 7 9 1 5
            6 9 1 5 4 8 7 3 2
            7 5 2 9 1 3 8 4 6
9 4 8 1 3 6 2 7 5 3 9 1 6 8 4 1 7 2 9 3 5
6 5 1 7 2 9 4 3 8 7 5 6 1 2 9 5 3 6 4 8 7
3 7 2 8 4 5 1 6 9 4 8 2 3 5 7 8 4 9 2 1 6
7 8 3 9 5 1 6 2 4        8 7 1 3 6 4 5 9 2
2 1 4 6 8 3 9 5 7        4 9 6 2 5 1 8 7 3
5 9 6 2 7 4 3 8 1        5 3 2 7 9 8 6 4 1
4 6 7 5 1 2 8 9 3        9 1 5 6 8 7 3 2 4
1 2 5 3 9 8 7 4 6        7 6 8 4 2 3 1 5 9
8 3 9 4 6 7 5 1 2        2 4 3 9 1 5 7 6 8
```

10. The word ladder
These are just examples:
A: hear—sound—music—emotion—anger—fight
B: storm—lightning—electricity—energy—food—rice
C: flask—drink—water—river—fish—net
D: child—school—book—paper—tree—forest

11. Hungry lion
1. Take off your shirt and try to throw it over the candle to douse it.
2. Stop imagining being in that situation.
3. It is a trained circus lion, and when you sing "happy birthday" it will walk over to the candle and blow it out.

12. Shooting arrows
A: 14
B: 43
C: 11
D: Carla 23

13. Scrambled sentences
A: Daily exercises can boost memory and concentration skills
B: Your brain uses about as much energy as a refrigerator light
C: No matter how ticklish you might be you can't tickle yourself
D: Learning to play a musical instrument improves spatial reasoning
E: Physical exercise and a good diet maintains brain health
F: Emotionally intense events produce vivid memories
G: Social skills depend on the awareness of what others are feeling

15. Stacking mosaic tiles
B

16. Quick-fire riddles
A: Only once. After that you would be subtracting from 20.
B: Chalkboard/blackboard
C: Your name

17. Krazy Kakuro
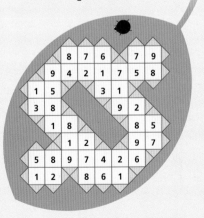

18. Spot the errors
A: The baby **wailed** throughout the church service
B: He was an **accessory** to the crime
C: They **accommodated** us really well during our holidays
D: Philip was definitely **unaccustomed** to public speaking
E: The weather looks very **changeable**
F: The teacher was very **disappointed**
G: The television was cheap but came without a **guarantee**

20. Complete the cube
C and E

21. Colored squares
Same. It may look as if the 2 arms of the "X" use different shades of pink, but in fact the whole "X" only uses a single color.

Painters have long known that the way a color looks in a painting is affected not only by the actual shade of the color itself, but also by the colors that surround it.

22. Shopping task
Tops: x 1 (= $48.50)
Skirts: x 3 (= $67.50)
Socks: x 4 (= $18)
Belt: x 3 (= $12.90)
(Total = $146.90)

24. Build the bird
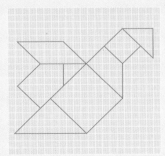

25. Suitor challenge
The successful suitor simply asked the daughter to walk over to where he stood and to touch his hand!

26. Fitting jigsaw pieces
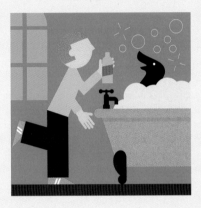

27. The shortest route

Useful websites

General

NewScientist
www.newscientist.com/topic/brain
For more information and the latest
research into how the brain works

Memory techniques

www.youramazingbrain.org/yourmemory

www.mindtools.com

www.buildyourmemory.com

www.changingminds.org/techniques/
memory/peg

Mind maps and Tony Buzan
www.buzanworld.com

The World Memory Championships
www.worldmemorychampionships.com

More puzzles and exercises

www.stetson.edu/~efriedma/puzzle
For a huge range of puzzles

Visual reasoning and spatial awareness

www.geocities.com/CapeCanaveral/
Lab/8972/

www.sharpbrains.com

Think creatively

www.cul.co.uk/creative/puzzles.htm

www.learning-tree.org.uk

Creative Problem Solving Institute
Creative Education Foundation
www.mycoted.com

Numerical reasoning

www.cut-the-knot.com

www.jimloy.com
For more numerical riddles

www.krazydad.com
For more Sudoku puzzles

www.riddles.com
For further creative conundrums

www.visualmathlearning.com

Verbal reasoning

www.puzzlechoice.com
For crosswords, word searches,
and word play games

www.wordplays.com
For more verbal games

Mind-body

Acupuncture

American Academy of Medical
Acupuncture
www.medicalacupuncture.org
Learn about acupuncture and how
to find an acupuncturist

Meditation

International Meditation Center–USA
internationalmeditationcentre.org/usa
For more information on meditation

Stress

American Institute of Stress
www.stress.org
Advice on symptoms, treatment, and
prevention

T'ai Chi

Taoist T'ai Chi Society of the
United States of America
www.usa.taoist.org
Part of the International Taoist T'ai Chi
Society; for more information on T'ai
Chi, including where to find a teacher in
the US

Yoga

Yoga Alliance
www.yogaalliance.org
Find a certified yoga teacher in the US

Further reading

Introduction to the brain

The Rough Guide to the Brain by Barry Gibb (Rough Guides), 2007

The Private Life of the Brain by Susan Greenfield (Wiley), 2000

The Human Brain: A Guided Tour by Susan Greenfield (Basic Books), 1998

Memory

Use Your Memory: Understand Your Mind to Improve Your Memory and Mental Power by Tony Buzan (BBC Active), 2006

How to Develop a Brilliant Memory Week by Week: 52 Proven Ways to Enhance Your Memory Skills by Dominic O'Brien (Duncan Baird Publishers), 2005

Your Memory: How It Works and How to Improve It by Kenneth L. Higbee (Da Capo Press), 2001

Visual reasoning and spatial awareness

Visual and Spatial Analysis: Advances in Data Mining, Reasoning, and Problem Solving by Boris Kovale-chuk & James Schwing (Springer), 2005

Mensa Mighty Visual Puzzles: Over 300 Puzzles To Test Your Powers Of Reasoning by John Bremner (Carlton Books Ltd), 1997

Near and Far at the Beach: Learning Spatial Awareness Concepts (Math for the Real World: Early Emergent) by Amanda Boyd (Rosen Publishing Group), 2008

Creativity

This is Your Brain on Music: Understanding a Human Obsession by Daniel J. Levitin (Atlantic Books), 2008

Mind Mapping: Kickstart Your Creativity and Transform Your Life (Buzan Bites) by Tony Buzan (BBC Active), 2006

The Power of Creative Intelligence by Tony Buzan (Thorsons), 2001

How to Have Creative Ideas: 62 Exercises to Develop the Mind by Edward De Bono (Vermilion), 2007

Thinkertoys: A Handbook of Creative-Thinking Techniques by Michael Michalko (Ten Speed Press), 2006

Numerical reasoning

Mensa Challenge Your Brain Math and Logic Puzzles (Official Mensa Puzzle Book) by Dave Tuller & Michael Rios (Sterling), 2006

Train Your Brain by Ryuta Kawashima (Kumon Publishing), 2008

Testing Series: How to Pass Numerical Reasoning Tests: A Step-by-step Guide to Learning the Basic Skills by Heidi Smith (Kogan Page), 2003

Verbal reasoning

The Power of Verbal Intelligence: 10 Ways to Tap into Your Verbal Genius by Tony Buzan (Thorsons), 2002

Practice Tests for Critical Verbal Reasoning by Peter Rhodes (Hodder Arnold), 2006

Verbal Reasoning: Challenge Tests by Stephen McConkey (Learning Together), 2007

Mind-body connection

How the Body Shapes the Mind by Shaun Gallagher (Oxford University Press), 2006

The Feeling of What Happens: Body, Emotion and the Making of Consciousness by Antonio R. Damasio (Harvest), 2000

The Yoga Bible: The Definitive Guide to Yoga Postures by Christina Brown (Walking Stick Press), 2003

Finding the Still Point: A Beginner's Guide to Zen Meditation by John Daido Loori (Shambhala Publications Inc), 2007

1001 Ways to Relax by Susannah Marriott (DK Publishing), 2008

Final workout (puzzles)

The Buzan Study Skills Handbook: The Shortcut to Success in Your Studies with Mind Mapping, Speed Reading and Winning Memory Techniques by Tony Buzan (BBC Active), 2006

The Big Book of Mind-bending Puzzles (Official Mensa Puzzle Book) by Terry H. Stickels (Sterling), 2006

The 10-Minute Brain Workout by Gareth Moore (Michael O'Mara Books Ltd), 2006

Will Shorts Presents KenKen Easy to Hard: 100 Logic Puzzles That Make You Smarter by Tetsuya Miyamoto (St. Martin's Griffin), 2008

Other interesting reading

The Man Who Mistook His Wife for a Hat by Oliver Sacks (Simon & Schuster), 1986

Six Thinking Hats by Edward de Bono (Back Bay Books), 2000

Emotional Intelligence: Why it Can Matter More Than IQ by Daniel Goleman (Bantam Books), 1996

The Lost Cause: An Analysis of Causation and the Mind-body Problem by Celia Green (Oxford Forum), 2003

Teach Yourself Training Your Brain by Simon Wootton & Terry Horne (McGraw-Hill), 2007

Phantoms in the Brain: Human Nature and the Architecture of the Mind by V.S. Ramachandran & Sandra Blakeslee (Fourth Estate Ltd.), 1999

Index

About the Authors

James Harrison

Harrison is a writer and editor. He cowrote *The Buzan Study Skills Handbook* (BBC Active, 2006), and was editorial consultant on *How to Be Confident Using the Power of NLP* (Prentice Hall Life, 2008) and *How to Help Your Child Succeed At School* (Prentice Hall Life, 2007). Harrison edited *Natural Choice* (Orbis), which explored complementary therapies for mind-body-spirit. He is currently working on a series of "Mind Set" books by Tony Buzan (BBC Active), which include titles on Mind Mapping, memory boosting and speed reading.

Mike Hobbs

Mike is an author, journalist, and copywriter. He has written nine books, including *The Big Challenge: Working Your Way To Health* (BBC Books, 2005) and *Easy PC* (Right Way, 2008). In addition, he has ghostwritten six more on subjects as diverse as soccer, pop music, and sex changes. His journalism has been published in the *Daily Telegraph*, the *Financial Times*, the *Guardian*, the *Independent*, *Time Out,* and the *Independent on Sunday*. Through his company, Westword, he has written marketing and public relations material for 20 years.

Acknowledgments

Authors' acknowledgments

This was a team effort in which we were merely players, so firstly we'd like to thank Peggy Vance for championing the project and for her enthusiastic support throughout. Our gratitude also goes to Suhel Ahmed and Charlotte Seymour for the tough task of marrying the words and design, and to Helen Murray, Penny Warren, and Liz Sephton for their calm overseeing. Our particular thanks also to Keith Hagan, who has created extremely eye-catching illustrations to make *Brain Training* really stand out. Thanks also to Phil Chambers for his knowledgeable and helpful advice. A heartfelt thanks to Tony Buzan for being an inspiration and showing that there are no limits to the amazing brain and that it is possible to create a manual for it!

Of course, finally a big thank you to our families (Joanna Harrison, Katie, Hugo, and Louise; Maureen Hobbs, Anna, Jack, and Elliott) for watching us both live in "puzzlesville," putting up with endless quizzes—and inadvertently training their brains in the process.

Publisher's acknowledgments

DK Publishing would like to thank Sue Bosanko for the index and Angela Baynham for proofreading in such a short amount of time. Also, many thanks to Matilda Gollon, Felicity Blackshaw, and Clementine Beauvais for editorial assistance, and Jennifer Murray and Ivy Fisher for checking the puzzles.

We would like to thank the following people/websites for providing access to their puzzles and exercises:

www.umapalata.com for "Building fences," p.21 and "Build the bird," p.170.

www.stetson.edu/~efriedma/color/ for "Numerical jigsaw," p.24, "Color mazes," p.26.

www.sharpbrains.com for "Cake for eight," p.52, "Quick-speed counting," p.53.

www.geocities.com/CapeCanaveral/Lab/8972 for "Largest circle," p.53, "Straight or crooked?", p.54, "Largest parcel," p.54, "The vanishing area," p.60.

www.mycoted.com for "A perfect circle?", p.21, "Speed reading," p.23, "Manhole covers," p.25, "Drinking glasses," p.73, "The elder twin," p73, "The swimmer in the forest," p.73, "Crossing the bridge," p.73, "Lateral thinking," p.78, "Original answers," p.84, "Strange detour," p.88, "Bottled money," p.88, "Separated at birth?", p.89, "Push that car," p.89, "Triangle ratio," p.105, "Chasing cars," p.120.

Oh Teik Bin for "Creative conundrums," pp.86–87, "The fatal flash," p.88, "Lax borders," p.88.

www.riddles.com for "Enough fish," p.72, "Newspaper divider," p.89, "Nail on the tree," p.89.

www.cul.co.uk/creative/puzzles.htm for "The hidden story," p.70, "Horsing around," p.72.

Brian Clegg (*Instant Brainpower*, Kogan Page Ltd, 1999) for "Summer job," p.136.

www.learning-tree.org.uk for "Matchstick mayhem," pp.00–03 and p.104.

www.efinancialcareers.co.uk for "Keen student," p.101, "Computer sales," p.103.

www.cut-the-knot.com for "The broken calculator," p.104.

www.krazydad.com for "Kakuro," pp.112–113 and p.167.

www.jimloy.com for "The famous 3 doors conundrum," p.121.

www.visualmathslearning.com for "The shortest route," p.104 and p.171.